Feel Great,
Be Beautiful
Over 40!

Feel Great, Be Beautiful Over 40!

By Lillian Müller and John Coleman

with Jill Alison Ganon

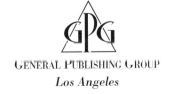

GPG

GENERAL PUBLISHING GROUP

Los Angeles

Publisher: W. Quay Hays

Art Director: Susan Anson

Managing Editor: Peter Hoffman

Copy Editor: Robin Quinn

Production Director: Nadeen Torio

Color and Prepress Director: Gaston Moraga

All photos & art work © 1995 by Lillian Müller, except cover Bill Dobbins, page 12 Richard Fegli, page 18, 58, 82, 200, back cover
Jan Rozenbergs, page 118 Mindas, page 136 Per Ervik, page 224 Barbro Fauski Steinde, page 160 Morten Quale, page 170 unknown

For information:
General Publishing Group, Inc.
2701 Ocean Park Boulevard
Santa Monica, CA 90405

Library of Congress Catalog Card Number 95-078489

ISBN: 1-881649-61-X

Printed in the USA
10 9 8 7 6 5 4 3 2 1

General Publishing Group
Los Angeles

Table of Contents

FOREWORD **9**

INTRODUCTION **13**

CHAPTER ONE / Healthy Food Choices **19**

CHAPTER TWO / Food Combining **59**

CHAPTER THREE / The Body Under Siege **83**

CHAPTER FOUR / Recipes **105**

CHAPTER FIVE / My Pregnancy Experience **119**

CHAPTER SIX / Holistic Awakening:

        Fasting, Diets & Internal Cleansing **137**

CHAPTER SEVEN / The Importance of Exercise and Fitness **161**

CHAPTER EIGHT / Timeless Beauty Tips **171**

CHAPTER NINE / Aging Reversed **201**

CHAPTER TEN / Thinking, Spirituality and Attitude **225**

SUGGESTED READINGS **233**

INDEX **235**

To Alice Angelica Müller Coleman

Thank your our Darling Daughter for teaching us unconditional Love
and for giving us the most fulfilling moments of our lives . . . .
You are our Angel for all Eternity

––––––––

Acknowledgments

Laura Hart and Sky Redlove—Without their guidance and support,
I would never have gotten to this point!

Erin and Gene Stanlie—Their great wisdom, teaching and inspiration set me
on the road to optmal health.

Mario daSilvo—Thank you to the man who showed me how to work out
in the gym and to have fun doing it!

Special thanks to Hugh Hefner, Bruno Bernard, Lily Cavell,
and my family in Norway for all their love and support.

—Lillian Müller

Thanks to Kristi Scheidenhelm for being far more than a patient typist.

Thanks to H.E. Woolsey, Michael Franz, Alan Krieger, Tim Hamilton, Ken Medlock, George Topps,
Mike Egan, Ken Johnson, Nick Mariano, Jack Scalia and Tom O'Reilly for help in times of need.

Thanks to Jill Ganon for her excellent help, to Peter Hoffman, a wonderful, editor,
to W. Quay Hays and Sharon Hays for their great help and vision and to all the people at
General Publishing Group who contributed to the project.

Of course, special thanks to our families.

—John Coleman

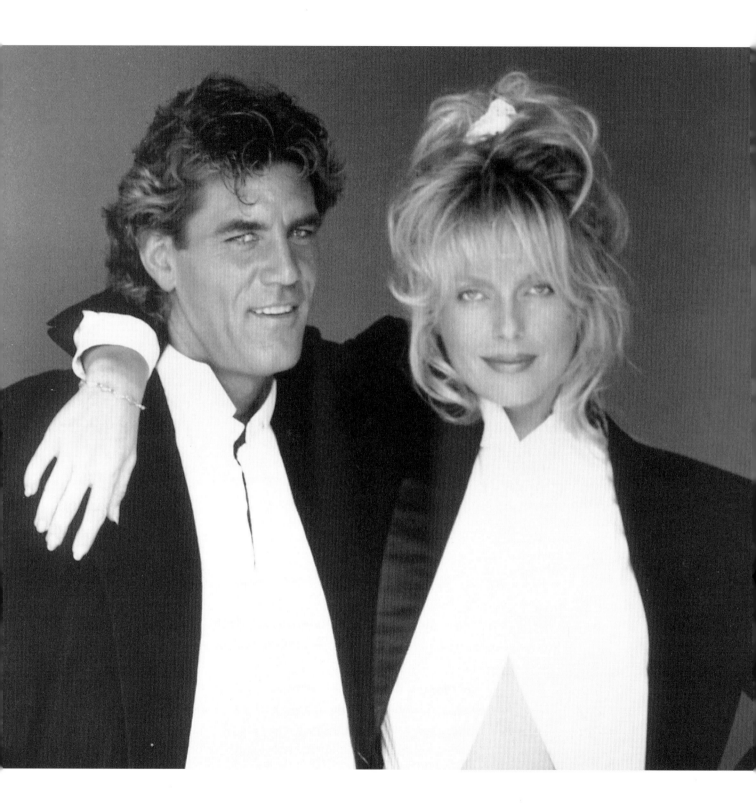

Foreword

If you were to sit down to dinner with Lillian, it is unlikely that you would leave the table without some reexamination of your eating habits. You might not push away your prime rib to share her vegetable plate, but the odds are good that you'd think twice about what to order the next time. When I met Lillian, I had already done a fair amount of investigation into nutrition. I was always active and athletic, and while you could accurately say I had a casual approach to diet, I was not uninformed.

From the beginning, Lillian and I did battle about our differing degrees of dedication to healthy eating. Certainly, nothing about Lillian's approach to diet could be called casual. And the payoff for all her vigilance was obvious. Beyond her beauty was a kind of glowing health more typically associated with women half her age. I recognized the need to make a commitment to healthier eating that would be realistic for me. But I firmly believed my moderate commitment would also show results. I structured my nutritional program with the intention of following it five days a week and the understanding that I'd feel satisfied with four. In six weeks, I had lost twenty-six pounds and I felt remarkably energetic. Beyond the simple satisfaction of having made improvements on my body, I was enjoying an exceptional sense of well-being. It was fantastic to eat as much as I wanted with no thought of "dieting." I found that I was not the only one benefiting from Lillian's years of study. Many of her friends were losing weight and growing more fit by revising their eating habits. None of us was a match for Lillian's level of commitment and yet the health improvements for all of us were significant. I began to talk to Lillian about putting her thoughts about health and nutrition down on paper. She protested that people would not follow the rigorous program she had outlined for herself. I argued that they would benefit from any degree of commitment to a healthier way of living. We started taking notes and the rest, as they say, is *Feel Great, Be Beautiful Over Forty!*

This is a book for anyone who wants to make informed choices about health. It will be of particular interest to the forty-something woman who is interested in making the kind of commitment to herself that will result in her looking and feeling great when she's an eighty-something woman. This is not a diet book, though it will help you to lose weight. It is not a self-improvement book, though it will empower you in your day-to-day life. This is a book about nutrition and lifestyle and it is filled with information about how to make healthful choices. For me, the rules of the game are very simple. By making informed decisions about what I eat each day, I choose to become more fit and energetic. And what about slipping back to old eating habits? That too is a choice with an all too predictable consequence: bloat, weight gain, energy loss, heavy feeling, irritability and wrinkles. I know that if I eat poorly, I'll have to pay the price: a tendency to gain weight and an unmistakable decline in energy. But what I've learned from Lillian is how to recover. And that is a gift available to anyone who is prepared to spend some time with this book.

There is no one way to eat properly. Everyone needs to tailor a program to his or her own lifestyle. But the bottom line is that the information in this book will provide you with a great place to start. The mirror doesn't lie, and I have seen fine lines in my face diminish in three to five days of healthy eating. I have seen the results in friends and associates of Lillian's who have reported immediate improvement to diagnosed conditions as varied as digestive ailments, eye strain and severe acne.

If you review this book carefully, I have no doubt that you will employ it at least occasionally. Even using it two days a week will provide a meaningful improvement in your diet. Spread out over twenty, forty or sixty years, it will make a gigantic difference in your life. Whether you are looking for a new lease on life or are simply a casual inquirer, this book will give you the tools to improve your health. Your body will thank you for using them.

—*John Coleman*

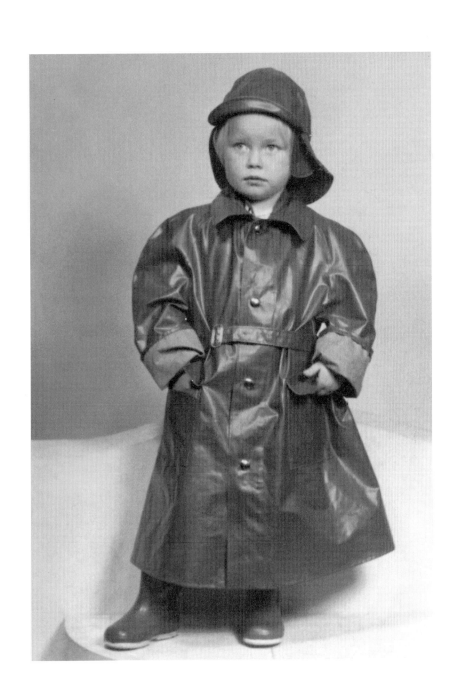

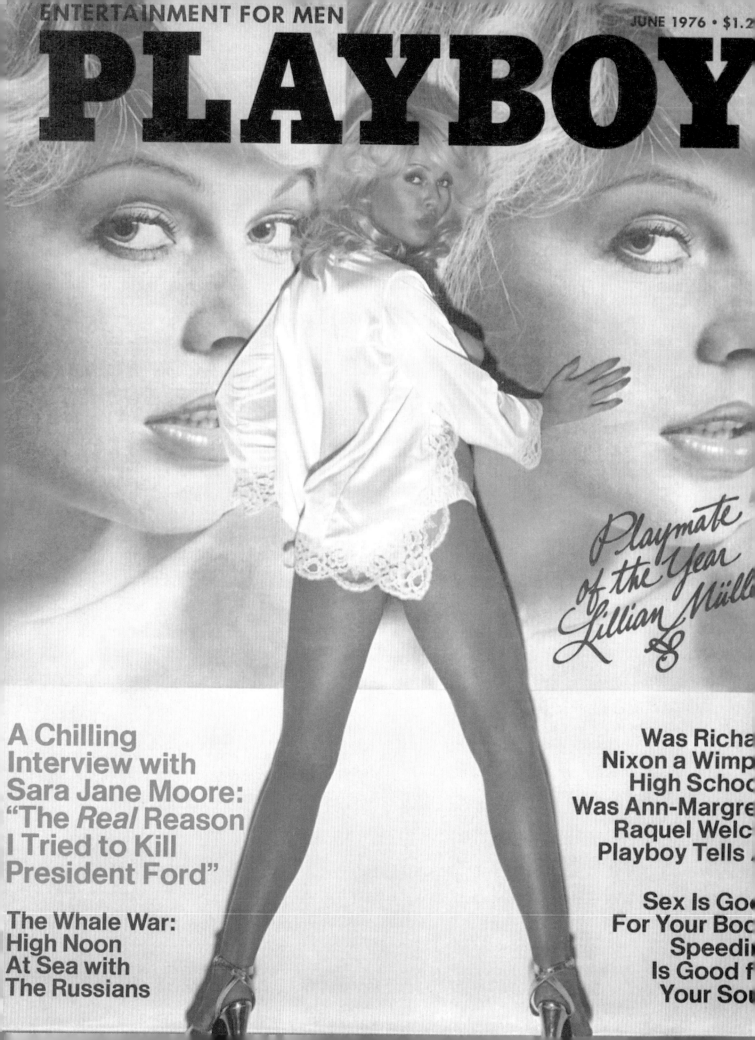

ENTERTAINMENT FOR MEN

JUNE 1976 • $1.2

PLAYBOY

*Playmate
of the Year
Lillian Müll*

**A Chilling
Interview with
Sara Jane Moore:
"The *Real* Reason
I Tried to Kill
President Ford"**

**The Whale War:
High Noon
At Sea with
The Russians**

**Was Richa
Nixon a Wimp
High Schoo
Was Ann-Margre
Raquel Welc
Playboy Tells**

**Sex Is Goo
For Your Boc
Speedin
Is Good f
Your Sou**

Introduction

My first contact with America was a sweet one. Every Christmas for as far back as I can remember, my father's two sisters sent us Christmas cards filled with Wrigley's chewing gum. America seemed impossibly far away from my village in Norway, and I loved my aunts, Ruth and Mabel, for sending us this incredible Christmas treat. My mother's sister Sonja also lived in America and she too sent candy that always arrived a few days before Christmas. There were caramel lollipops and marshmallows and thick Hershey bars with almonds that were my absolute favorite.

By the time I was nine, my love affair with America had moved beyond holiday sweets to include a complete infatuation with American movie stars. I bought chewing gum and candies that came with movie star trading cards. All the girls in the neighborhood would get together to trade our precious cards, and we would sit for hours, staring at our idols, talking about them, and dreaming up improbable futures for ourselves. My favorite star was Raquel Welch. I would sit, mesmerized, in front of the television, waiting for her to appear in the Lux soap commercial. She was a goddess to me and I wondered how an actual human being could look so divine. (And she still looks incredible almost thirty years later!)

But dreaming about movie stars while visiting the bakery every afternoon was a no-win situation. By my second year in high school, I had become quite chubby. My mother would tease me about ending up like my father's sisters, with their thick legs and ankles. My mother's long, graceful legs seemed much more in keeping with my ideal of beauty. I remember wishing she would just empty the house of all those tempting fresh-baked goodies. Somehow, I found the resolve to stop eating unlimited cake and ice cream and became thin again. Even though my figure still lacked the womanly curves I was hoping for, I figured it was better to be thin without curves than fat and still have no curves!

In the summer before my eighteenth birthday, I changed from an awkward, insecure teenager into a curvy and increasingly confident woman. For the first time, I was receiving attention from the opposite sex and it felt wonderful. In the following couple of years I became a finalist in the Miss Norway pageant and other beauty contests. At the age of 22, I had become a successful model in London. I was discovered by *Playboy* and suddenly the improbable future I dreamed of as a child was becoming reality. My successful centerfold led to my selection as Playmate of the Year and a long-standing relationship with *Playboy*.

But the challenges of adapting to my new life in America sent me running back to an old friend: food. I tried to eat away my nervousness and succeeded only in gaining unwanted pounds and additional anxiety. I now know that this experience is something I share with many women. We've all looked to food for non-threatening, unconditional support in time of need. But at the time, I felt guilty and secretive and very much alone. Why, if things were so good for me, was I feeling so bad? What was missing? As I write this, with the buffer of many years tempering my perspective, I know with absolute certainty that the missing ingredient was good health. How important is good health? We drink toasts to it. We wish it to our friends. We pray for it for our babies even before they're born. We mourn its loss with deepest regret. But how much work are we willing to do in pursuit of superior health? Years of study and experimentation with diet and exercise have given me my answer: I am willing to work damn hard. Granted, my modeling and acting careers put a premium on how I look, but my personal commitment to successful nutrition and holistic health practices puts a premium on how I feel. And feeling great is the secret to a "long run" in any career. I am the first to admit that my commitment is extreme, but with even a modest commitment the benefits of healthy living will begin to reveal themselves.

To have a total understanding of your health, you must view it from a number of related perspectives. A house can be viewed from either the front, sides, back or above. Each perspective is useful but incomplete. The information from several individualized perspectives must be integrated into a whole in order to truly view the house. Similarly, health is a series of related variables that are completely interdependent:

If one aspect of health is out of balance, the extraordinary machine that is your body will suffer.

What you eat and drink

When you eat and drink

How you combine what you eat and drink

How you exercise

What you breathe

How you think

We all share a natural tendency to focus upon those aspects of our lives that we believe to be successful. But what about the mother who follows a rigorously "healthy" diet and then fails to exercise; or the attorney who runs several miles each day but stresses out constantly over her work? In reality, while these individuals may view themselves as being extremely virtuous, they are out of balance. Once again, look at the world around you. Your car has an engine, tires, transmission, steering, fuel pump, etc. If any one of these elements is faulty, the car will not operate very long or go very far. Your body is also a machine. The heart and organs are its engine. The brain is its computer and the communications director of the nervous system. The food you put in your mouth is its fuel. The better the fuel, the better the engine will run and the more efficiently it will perform. Efficient performance is another way of describing the greatest gift we have to offer ourselves and our families: the gift of superior health. Unfortunately, if one aspect of health is out of balance, the extraordinary machine that is your body will suffer. This may manifest as kidney stones, gall stones, heart attack, liver problems, cancer or depression. When one of the body's functions is blocked, its operation shuts down and the whole system suffers. For example, if you were to break a leg and find it difficult to exercise, your body would burn fewer calories. Were you to continue to consume the same foods in the same quantities, weight gain would be inevitable. There would be loss of muscle tone, and your liver and kidneys would have to work harder to rid the body of toxins normally eliminated during exercise. Toxins would collect in the skin and hair, showing their unfortunate aging effects relatively quickly. Lack of exercise compounded by overeating would begin to sap you of motivation and happiness. The lesson is clear: The continued neglect of even one aspect of your health can eventually affect not only your body, but your mind and feelings as well. In other words, deprived of balance, the machine begins to break down. So what can you do?

Fortunately, this machine of ours is wonderfully responsive to good treatment. If you are a relatively healthy person, a week-long juice fast will begin to alleviate the accumulated effects of many toxins. There will be a dramatic improvement to the appearance of the skin, including a reduction of fine lines and wrinkles. Energy will be much enhanced, leading to greater vitality and the likelihood of increased social activity which in turn has its own rewards.

The human body is the only machine for which there are no spare parts.

Hermann M. Biggs

(1859 - 1923)

As I began to go over the years of notes that would eventually become this book, I realized that I was able to break down the nutritional information into three primary components:

- *The type of food/fuel you consume:* This is the obvious starting point. The better you eat, the more efficiently you'll function. I am happy to offer you a broad range of delicious, energy-giving food that you can choose to make readily available.

- *The importance of appropriate food combinations:* Once you've made the commitment to choosing healthy foods, you must learn how to successfully combine them for maximum energy efficiency.

- *The debilitating effects of mucus-producing foods:* A diet free of mucus-producing foods is unquestionably the healthiest way to go. Mucus collects throughout our bodies, slowly inhibiting our natural vitality. Many of our ailments can be addressed by reducing or eliminating mucus in our diets.

My path to a healthier life began with tentative steps toward improved nutrition. But it wasn't long before I learned that food was only one component of a complete reexamination of my life. In addition to nutritional enlightenment, my path to improved health was guided by numerous physical, spiritual and mental considerations. *Feel Great, Be Beautiful Over 40!* is my opportunity to share with you much of what I have learned. As a woman who has spent years in a business that puts a premium on beauty, I can tell you without hesitation what makes a woman truly beautiful. It isn't her age, or her measurements, or how well she makes up her face; it is her health. And glowing, energetic good health is a gift only you can give yourself.

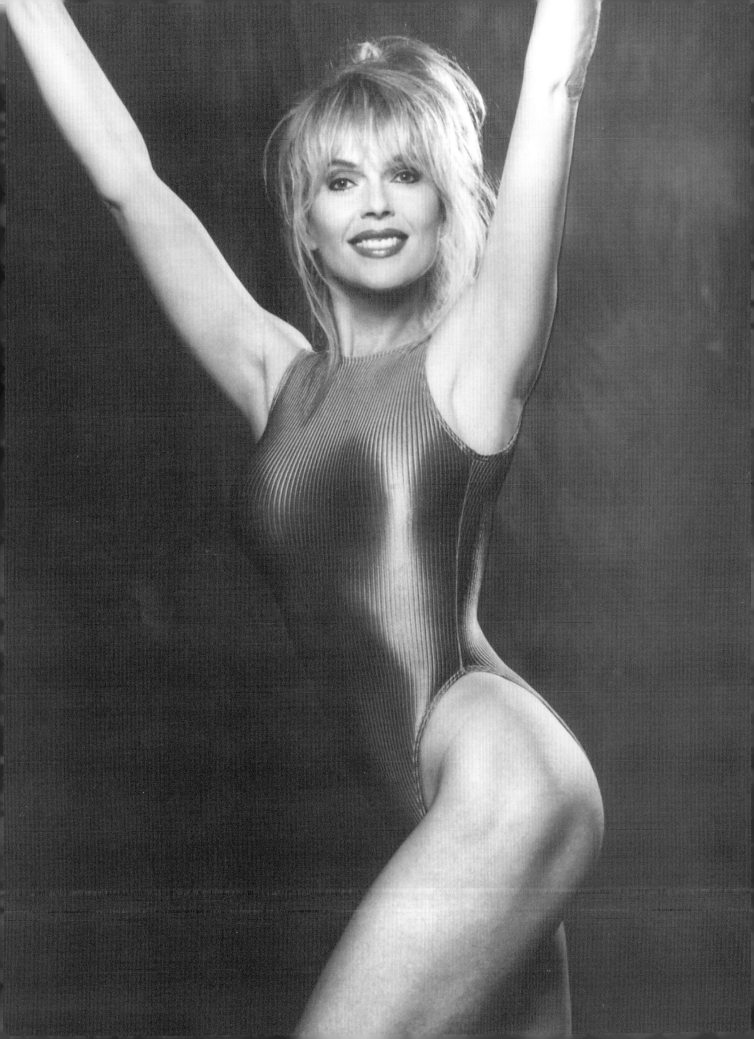

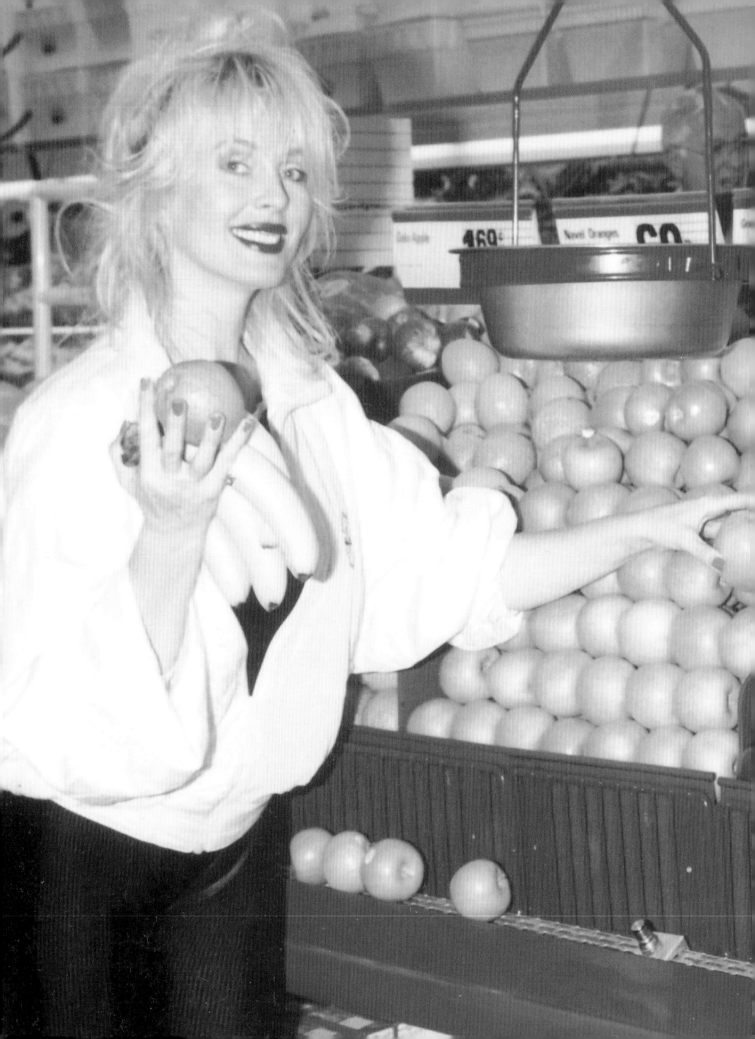

CHAPTER ONE

Healthy Food Choices

People should be able to make educated choices about something as important as their health. Unfortunately, the average person has no idea what constitutes a good diet. Yet informed choice is the single most empowering aspect of our lives. If a well-educated person chooses to eat an unhealthy diet, that is her choice. If an uninformed person does so, that is quite another thing.

Every day we are bombarded with information that glorifies the typical, unhealthy diet. You cannot drive down the street, watch television or read a magazine without having your appetite courted by the multi-billion-dollar food industry. The problem is that even as our society reexamines its eating habits, we fail to go beyond a surface appraisal. Everyone should know the truth about the many unhealthy and destructive foods that we consume today. Sometimes these foods have been part of our diets for so many generations that their use has become a part of our very lives. We may order a big steak to celebrate a business deal or send giant boxes of chocolates to our sweethearts. Isn't it ironic that these unhealthy foods have come to symbolize our successes and represent our love?

As you consider a new way of eating, it is important to realize that in addition to Madison Avenue, your eating habits have been ingrained into the culture for generations. It is important to be realistic in your expectations of yourself. Whether you "live to eat" or "eat to live," food will always

Give yourself a break!
Don't beat yourself up if you can't resist
the occasional french fry.

be an integral part of your life. Making an effective change in your eating habits takes time, effort and, most of all, desire. Don't expect to do it all at once. Remember, this is not a "diet." It is a way of living. The most important thing you can do for yourself at this point is to take pleasure and pride in anything you are doing to improve your health. Almost anyone can forego junk food for a week to squeeze into a sexy dress, but making a deliberate commitment to changing your lifelong eating habits is another matter entirely. Give yourself a break! Don't beat yourself up if you can't resist the occasional french fry. Remember, you're on your way. In this chapter, we're going to look at a broad range of food choices. To begin, I'd like to explain the particulars of my personal food program which may be of help as you begin to develop your own.

My Food Philosophy

I prefer to make my own meals from fresh ingredients. If I eat out, I go to a vegetarian restaurant or a health food store deli where food is prepared in accordance with my own food needs. More people are beginning to acknowledge the impact of a good diet on their health, and it is becoming easier to find establishments that cater to those needs. This concept is very prevalent in Los Angeles and that is one of the reasons I prefer to live here.

When I first heard of a diet limited solely to raw vegetarian foods, I thought it was absurd. I was living a busy urban life in L.A., not sipping drinks from coconuts in some remote tropical paradise. But irrefutable evidence of the success of a vegetarian lifestyle stood before me.

My friend was in his sixties but did not look a day over forty. For over six years, he had been on a self-created raw vegetable diet. His skin was golden and radiant. His face was almost wrinkle-free, and his eyes were clear and beautiful. His hair was shiny and healthy. He had an optimistic and joyful attitude toward life. Though he had aged chronologically, he was young in every sense of the word.

I asked him if he ever went off his raw food diet and ate cooked vegetarian foods or so-called junk foods. "No way," he replied. "I feel so much energy and joy and strength, and I have such a feeling of lightness, it's almost like I can fly. I would never go off of it. It has totally changed my life. I run six miles a day and I'm never tired. I won't indulge in unhealthy food just to have that instant pleasure of tasting it. I know very well that after eating it I would not feel the way I feel now. I lived on unhealthy foods most of my life, and I never felt good. Now I feel incredible. I don't want to mess it up by going back to my old ways."

Safeguard the health of both body and soul.

Cleobulus

When I finally tried his diet, it worked similar wonders for me. They say that nothing succeeds like success and now I know why. The raw vegetarian diet takes an incredible commitment, and I don't expect everyone to pursue it, but it has been worth the effort for me.

Believe me when I tell you I have yet to attain total commitment. I can be extremely vulnerable to a pint of chocolate ice cream in the freezer. But I know I am at my best—spiritually, mentally and physically—when I stay on the vegetarian wagon. I have met many other people with similar outlooks and they always inspire me. We laugh and commiserate about our indulgences and applaud each other's success stories. But I know now that I will work at eating healthily for the rest of my life, and I'm excited about inspiring others to try it for themselves.

I believe "toxic waste" in our bodies is the reason for most sickness, and consequently, I follow a program of preventive medicine and I have not been ill or even taken a pill in over seventeen years. I am rarely ill. Toxins are created by negative emotions, pollution, dangerous food additives, environmental chemicals, unhealthy diet or lack of proper elimination. When you change your lifestyle for the better, you feel well again in a relatively short amount of time. Once in a while I catch a cold or have a nagging pain somewhere in my body. Perhaps I feel stressed or tired. In those cases, I try to listen to my body and watch my lifestyle more carefully. I concentrate on drinking plenty of juices and purified water, and eat plenty of fresh fruits and salads. That diet always seems to cure me of any minor ailment, and I am back to normal within a couple of days. I prefer to maintain a low-fat, low-protein, high-carbohydrate diet. I know that I function best on lots of fresh fruits and their juices, dried fruits and raw, unsalted nuts. I also consume raw and steamed fresh vegetables and their juices, baked potatoes and yams and a small amount of whole grain breads and cereals, supplemented by limited quantities of soy milk and tofu products. Once in a while I put raw, unsalted butter on my toast or steamed vegetables. Believe me, I know this sounds extreme to most people, but you will be amazed at how quickly your body will respond to being treated this well.

Think of the typical American sandwich: processed meats on white bread supplemented with high fat mayonnaise. This is a perfect example of bad food combining. But consider this: a "vegetarian sandwich" with whole grain bread or toast, loaded with avocado, tomato, cucumber and sprouts. Add a little unsalted soy mayonnaise and fresh ground pepper and you have a delicious lunch. Popular condiments and other seasoning agents contain a vast array of undesirable substances, both natural and synthetic, which I try

The road to healthy eating
can have many rest stops along the way.
It is okay to start the journey
with a modest goal.

to avoid. Consequently, I use the purest forms of ketchup, mustard and dry herbal flavoring powders I can find. With a little research and a lot of taste testing, I have managed to restrict my intake of salt and sugar, as well as other common additives. I put natural ketchup on my baked potato strips or steamed vegetables. Jensen's Dry Vegetable Seasoning is a favorite on sandwiches.

Vegeburgers, soy burgers and soy hot dogs sound like healthy products, but they contain salt in a quantity I consider unhealthy. When I eat them, I do so with this in mind, and know I will suffer unwanted consequences if I overindulge. Occasionally I snack on air-popped popcorn with a little sea salt or vegetable powder sprinkle.

The road to healthy eating can have many rest stops along the way. It is usually best to start the journey with a modest goal. Commit to a month of trading in your regular chips and munchies for some of the snacks I suggest on page 33. You'll be amazed at how successfully your taste buds adapt to restricted salt, fat and sugar. Many people report that after a month of restricted salt intake, heavily salted foods like chips and luncheon meats are distinctly unpleasant to eat. The lesson here is that if you make the initial effort, your body will do the rest!

My Personal Program

I maintain a diet of totally raw foods for long periods every year. This is the food program that provides me with the greatest levels of vitality and motivation. It is the raw unprocessed whole foods in the vegetarian diet that I recommend most. If you are one of the people who can never feel satisfied on a totally raw diet, I still hope you will stay away from all sugary, salty foods. Not everyone is willing to live on raw, "live" foods, but it works so wonderfully for me that I cannot resist recommending that you try it for yourself.

Think about it for a moment. If you are looking for a spark to jump start a renewed energy in your life, this might be your answer. I know it is one thing to refrain from chips and dip for a month and another thing entirely to limit yourself to raw fruits and vegetables for that long. Remember, I have been at this for many years and have worked myself up to this level of commitment. But let's say you've tried giving up your old salty snacks and find yourself munching quite contentedly on air-popped popcorn. Maybe you are ready to try a month-long raw foods program. Or perhaps you want to commit to several days a week or certain meals each day.

One way is to get yourself a notebook and keep a record of the foods you eat as well as your feelings throughout the month. This journal will be a

Once you become conscious of wanting *to make changes in your eating habits, keeping a food journal offers you the opportunity to tune in to highly motivating changes in your health, weight and mental outlook.*

very important tool in modifying your eating habits. How difficult or easy was the transition to raw foods? When did you most feel the urge to "cheat"? What sorts of foods did you crave? Which were the easiest to give up? What feelings sent you racing to the refrigerator or even the drive-through window? A month of accountability for your eating will speak volumes about how to change your eating habits.

After a month passes, read over your journal entries and judge for yourself. Did you have more energy? Did you begin to experience any of the feelings of well-being I have described? Are there changes, subtle or dramatic, to your body? Once you become conscious of *wanting* to make changes in your eating habits, keeping a food journal offers you the opportunity to tune in to highly motivating changes in your health, weight and mental outlook. I think you'll be pleasantly surprised by the available vitality you'll receive for your efforts. Don't make the mistake of thinking it is necessary to change to all raw meals immediately. I believe that if you stick to a vegetarian diet of both cooked and raw foods you will definitely feel much better. In Chapter Two, I explain in more depth the practicalities of food combining.

At this point, I think it is helpful to begin to consider some of the options along the road to healthier eating. While I rarely eat cooked foods

Out with the Old... In with the New!

Don't despair. There are are delicious, healthful alternatives to many of your traditional "comfort foods." Don't give up until you find the brand you enjoy. Believe me, it can be done.

OUT	IN
potato chips, cheese puffs	baked chips, popcorn (air popped)
high-fat ice cream	low-fat frozen yogurt or soy ice cream
sugary cookies	juice-sweetened cookies
hot dogs and hamburgers	soy dogs and vegeburgers
chocolate milk	carob-flavored rice milk and soy milk

now, when I started to change my diet, I transitioned with primarily cooked vegetarian dishes. Compared to a diet that included animal flesh products, dairy products and sugary and salty junk foods, my new vegetarian diet supplied me with optimum energy and nutrition.

Gradually, it is possible to increase your intake of raw foods until you find you are consuming a primarily raw food diet. This process allows you

To avoid sickness, eat less,
to prolong life, worry less.

Chu Hui Weng
in "Bulletin of the New York Academy of Medicine,"
1928 (F.H. Garrison)

to become acclimated to new things and avoids shocking your system. As many veterans of the diet wars know all too well, if you attempt to change everything too abruptly, you may abandon your new way of eating and backslide into your old ways.

Health and Happiness

Everyone hopes to get what they want out of life. Why? To be happy. What if you could have what you wanted, but it didn't make you happy? With poor health, no matter what you have, it is very difficult to be happy. It is hard to laugh with a stomachache, headache, flu or a more serious ailment like a heart condition. A totally healthy body will give you a clarity, lightness and joyfulness that will go far in supporting your personal quest for happiness.

Personal Observations

Fruits, nuts, raw vegetables and drinks made from them make me feel and look my best, so I adhere to that program as strictly as possible. I cannot ignore the fact that in addition to my strong desire to be as healthy as I can be, much of my livelihood has for many years been linked to my looking as good as I can. It is not hard to imagine the pressures on women in the entertainment field, and we all find different ways of coping with them. My coping mechanism is what some people might label an obsessive or fanatical commitment to my health. Many friends joke with me about how I bring my own condiments, or sometimes my own meals, to restaurants. But part of what led me to write this book was the realization that those same friends who tease me about the degree of my devotion to this diet have reaped its benefits by maintaining their own levels of commitment to healthier eating.

This situation is not black or white, but is very much a matter of degree. Many people who want to be healthy have little interest in maintaining a program as rigorously controlled as mine. But they find their own degree of commitment and experience and have their own wonderful success stories. Since it works for me, I stay on it. Believe me when I tell you there are many skeletons in my culinary closet! Cheese, Norwegian gravlax and rich, creamy ice cream still have a certain hold over me. Many Norwegian dishes such as sardines, cod and various cakes and cookies were a delicious staple of my diet as a child. When I visit Norway, my childhood treats are hard to resist. My family still laughs about the time I visited Norway during my pregnancy and stood in my mother's kitchen gnawing on sausages straight from the pot. "Oh, I'll just try one," I said to myself as I tasted my first sausage. Nine big links later, I had

Different foods make you
feel and look relatively better or worse,
depending on your reaction to them.

eaten enough to have fed the entire family. Of course, the salt made my ankles swell up like inner tubes and I refused to let anyone look at my feet for almost a week. But I have to confess, at that particular moment, those sausages were absolutely delicious! A bellyful of sausages notwithstanding, there is an obvious payoff when I control my cravings for these foods: avoiding the days of sluggishness that always follow a deviation from my regular routine.

Different foods make you feel and look relatively better or worse, depending on your reaction to them. I try to stay on an uncooked vegetarian diet four to five days a week. On the remaining days, I add some cooked vegetarian foods at mealtime, but almost never eat animal foods. Over the years I have gradually lost my appetite for most meat, fowl and seafood products. I used to crave them, especially when I was having PMS symptoms, and on occasion, I had quite a battle with myself to abstain from eating them. Now that I have been a vegetarian for many years, I am rarely tempted. If I do eat chicken or fish at a social gathering, I feel the disruption to my system for several days. After years of vigilance, my style of eating has at last become a habit, and I follow my guidelines routinely. I don't have to think about it unless I am tempted to eat "unhealthy" foods.

Cravings!

If you tend to experience particular food cravings over and over again, there may be help available in the form of homeopathic remedies.

Try **phosphorus** if your cravings are for salt, spicy foods and ice cream.

Sepia has provided relief to those who crave sour, bitter, pungent and spicy foods.

If you experience cravings for eggs, milk, sweets, salt and raw potatoes, your homeopath may decide to treat you with **calcarea carbonica**.

Lycopodium may be the answer for you if you become ravenously hungry right after a big meal.

Future Diet Directions

I am now at the point where I am trying to minimize grains and starches in my diet. My system has become very pure after years of good diet and cleansing, and it is very sensitive to any starchy foods. I still have occasional cravings, but I am slowly moving toward giving them up completely. Just as I stopped desiring concentrated protein foods from animal sources, so will I

I did not become a vegetarian for my health.
I did it for the health of the chickens.

Isaac Bashevis Singer (1904 - 91)

stop craving starchy foods.

I have no doubt that a diet of fresh fruits, dried fruits, raw nuts and seeds, and raw vegetables is the best diet for my personal well-being. You will have to research what works best in *your* case. I think the "diet" issue is very personal, and is certainly subject to as many emotional decisions as nutritional ones. Many people simply could not function well on a diet like mine, particularly in a cold climate. Whenever I travel to Norway or Minnesota on vacation, I crave more warm foods. My body seems to need it, to be asking

Healthy Snack Alternatives

Celery Boats — Fill celery sticks with nut butters or tofu spreads.

Jicama Sticks — Raw or marinated in lime juice with a pinch of sea salt.

Overripe Bananas — Peel and insert a stick before freezing in plastic for a healthy popsicle.

Trail Mix — Add powdered or flaked sea vegetables to enhance their mineral content.

Dried Fruits — Combine with nuts and seeds and eat the fruits first.

Fresh Fruits — Raw, as fruit kabobs, or blended into smoothies, with nuts and seeds for variation.

Popcorn — Air popped and flavored with garlic, chili powder, various salt-free herbal seasonings, ground pepper, brewer's yeast, or warm with a little raw butter melted over the top.

Chips — Unsalted whole grain corn, whole grain rice, or potato chips with natural salsa, preferably unsalted.

French Bakes — Slice raw potatoes into sticks and bake them in the oven (rather than french fry). Serve plain, with herbal sprinkles, natural ketchup or other salt-free sauces and condiments.

Baked Eggplant — Slice an eggplant into sticks or rounds, brush with olive oil and Bragg's Liquid Amino and bake until very light brown.

for more. Then I eat lots of hearty veggie stews and potatoes and whole grains. I also eat more nuts and seeds when I am there.

Now that you've had an opportunity to learn a little about my diet and how I came to develop it, I'd like you to look over the following lists of foods. They are broken down into food groups and are designed to ease your transition into healthier eating.

I am at the point where I typically follow the raw food regimen of

*Tell me what you eat and
I will tell you what you are.*

Anthelme Brillat-Savarin (1755 - 1826)

On the Road to Healthy Eating

The following food lists, designated at Levels 1, 2 and 3, will provide you with instant insight into the gradual process of improving your diet. Level 1 is appropriate for an individual who is in the initial stages of the transition to healthier eating. You will quickly see that Level 1 is the most inclusive of the three levels, as it includes non-vegetarian foods. Naturally, Level 1 eaters should seek to include any of the wonderful vegetarian foods from Levels 2 and 3.

LEVEL 1:
(Includes Levels 2 & 3)

- Organically grown chicken or turkey (raised on natural feed and free of hormones, steroids and antibiotics)
- Organically produced chicken eggs
- All natural dairy products (preferably raw)
- Fresh fish (from cold, less polluted waters)
- All foods derived from the above ingredients

LEVEL 2:
(Includes Cooked Foods)

- Steamed vegetable soups and stews
- Baked and broiled vegetables
- Baked potatoes, yams and sweet potatoes
- Hard squashes
- Air-popped popcorn with herb seasoning
- Stuffed potatoes (meatless/cheeseless)
- Baked french fries
- Chips—rice, potato or corn (preferably baked)
- Spaghetti and pasta (meatless)
- Whole grain breads
- Vegetarian sandwiches
- Whole grain cakes and cookies
- Meatless chili (homemade) and canned beans
- Homemade and canned vegetable soup
- Vegetarian burgers
- Soy products, including soy in its many forms as yogurts, milk, freezes, tofu, hot dogs, burgers, sausage, bacon, meatballs, cheese, etc.
- Brown rice, oatmeal, whole grain pancakes, cornbread, and other whole grain foods
- Meatless frozen foods available in health food stores
- Nut butters (roasted)
- Meatless tamales
- Fruit jams, unsweetened
- Ketchup, mustard and condiments (unsalted, sugar-free)
- Vegetable seasonings (no salt, unflavored, no additives)
- Bragg's Liquid Amino (salt substitute) and Jensen's Dry Vegetable Seasoning
- Other herbal salt substitutes
- Unsalted, sugar-free spaghetti sauce
- Garlic and onion powders
- Raw butter, cream and milk
- Raw milk cheeses
- Natural soda
- Soy milk, rice milk, amazake
- Curry seasoning, vegetarian bouillon for soups

LEVEL 3:
(Raw Foods)

- Raw fruits and raw vegetables
- Fresh-squeezed juices and smoothies, nut/seed "milks," herbal teas
- Fruit sorbets, raw nut/banana freezes
- Dried fruits
- Raw nut/seed butters, yogurt and cheese
- Raw sprouted seeds, beans or grains
- "Energy soup," guacamole, fresh salads
- Raw veggie sticks
- Raw carob powder, dehydrated "pies" and "cookies"
- Vegetable sushi, kelp, dulse, and sea vegetable seasonings

Food that is attractive to the eye
is somehow more appealing to the palate.

Level 3, supplemented with some foods from Level 2. But keep in mind that my road to healthy eating has been a long one with many twists and turns. These suggested food lists are not so rigidly constructed that some foods are permitted and some forbidden. There are hundreds of great tasting, healthy foods from which to choose. My program is not about "eating this" and "not eating that." Instead, it is meant to provide you with the opportunity to eat healthy foods most, if not all, of the time.

Successful Snacking

The digestive system works best when we are seated. Eat snacks sitting down instead of while standing, walking or lying down.

- Don't snack within two hours of bedtime. The body sleeps best on an empty stomach. You will sleep deeply and awaken refreshed. If, occasionally, you feel very hungry before bedtime, choose a snack that is easy to digest and low in fat.
- Arrange your foods in an attractive manner before you sit down to eat them. Food that is attractive to the eye is somehow more appealing to the palate. You might want to eat raw apples whole most of the time, but, for variety, you can also quarter apples and serve them on a plate with dried figs and raw nuts.
- Enjoy your snacks and don't feel guilty. Choose healthy foods that taste great to you.

Healthy Snacking

Once you start preparing healthier meals for yourself, it is still tempting to grab junk foods here and there when you are hungry and in a hurry. Many of the snacks listed here can be prepared and stored ahead of time. Cut up vegetables such as carrots, jicima, potatoes and celery and store them in a small amount of purified water in airtight containers in your refrigerator.

Sweet Alternatives

Human beings are universally attracted to sweets. Whether enjoying sugar cane or Belgian chocolates, children all over the world learn early on to appreciate sweet tastes. Fortunately, there are many delicious alternatives to refined sugar.

Date Sugar is made from ground, dried dates and has the same nutritional value as dates. It is very sweet and can be used in baked desserts in place of refined sugar. Simply add enough hot water to turn the date sugar into a

Supplement your whole grain breads and pastas with proper proportions of fresh fruits, vegetables, nuts, seeds, peas and beans.

thick syrup. I sprinkle date sugar on cereal and oatmeal or whenever I might be tempted to use refined sugar.

Fruit Juice Concentrates are fruit juices with most of the water removed. They are used in many commercially available prepared natural foods, such as cereal, cookies and syrups.

Maple Syrup has a unique, woodsy flavor. It causes blood sugar levels to fluctuate, but not as radically as syrups made from malted grains or refined sugar. Maple sugar, when available, is the concentrated, crystallized form of maple syrup.

Honey contains low levels of vitamins, pollen and certain enzymes. Dark honeys are richer in minerals, but light-colored honeys have a milder taste.

Barley Malt Syrup is a natural grain sweetener with a rich, malty flavor. It is made from soaked and sprouted barley or hot-air dried barley combined with water. This mixture is cooked into a thick, sweet syrup. It is absorbed by the body at a slower rate than refined sweeteners and has a more moderate effect on blood sugar levels.

Kick the (Soda) Can

A can of soda can contain as much as a whopping 16 teaspoons of sugar. Instead of reaching for "the real thing," try "bubbly" water and fruit juice. There are several juice-sweetened sodas on the market, or you can make your own by adding any 100% fruit juice to carbonated water. It is wonderfully refreshing and children love it.

Brown Rice Syrup is a mild sweetener usually made by combining cooked brown rice with sprouted barley. It has a more subtle flavor than barley malt syrup, but shares the same gentle effect on blood sugar levels. Rice syrup has the highest protein level of any natural sweetener and is an especially good choice for baking.

Candy Substitutes include dried, sulfur-less fruits of every variety, barley-sweetened bon-bons and many carob confections instead of chocolate.

The Chinese do not draw any distinction between food and medicine.

Lin Yutang (1895 - 1976)

Author, linguist in his essay "The Importance of Living"

Whole Grain Breads and Pastas

Whole grain breads and pastas are tasty alternatives to those products made from white, processed flour. White flour becomes pasty inside your body, forming a substance much like white glue, and has a tendency to make you constipated. White flour also has very low nutritional value, so it clogs the system without providing any nutritional benefits. Sprouted grains are much better for human digestion. When grains are sprouted, their starch is converted into sugar which can be assimilated by the body much more easily than starch.

Whole grains provide a good supply of fiber which is important in maintaining regular bowel movements. If your diet is deficient in fiber, the walls of your colon will not be "swept out" as often. This can result in constipation, bloating and other problems, such as an increased risk of colon cancer.

Sprouted grains provide vastly increased nutritional value over dried grains. Unprocessed grain retains nearly all of its vitamins and minerals, but the minute it is ground into flour or processed it begins to lose potency. Sprouted grains, on the other hand, are much better for you. I personally prefer to eat bread made from sprouted grains, without any added sugar, salt or preservatives. Sprouted grain bread is deliciously sweet, filling and full of nutrients.

Whole grain pastas, cereals, cakes and cookies not only taste wonderful, but they offer numerous other benefits. As you begin to experiment with healthy foods, you will find that eating a nutritional diet is just as satisfying to the palate as the average American diet of commercial high-fat, low-fiber foods. Have fun with it. You will find yourself reading labels and learning to analyze this information while shopping for food. Much of the food that is marketed to health conscious consumers actually contains many unhealthy additives.

Supplement your whole grain breads and pastas with proper proportions of fresh fruits, vegetables, nuts, seeds, peas and beans. Together, these foods will supply all your nutritional needs and plenty of fiber.

Exotic Grains

Quinoa: This small, super nutritious, disk-shaped seed was a staple of Inca culture. Quinoa, with generous amounts of B-complex, vitamin E, calcium, phosphorus and iron, is an almost complete protein source. It is easy to digest and ranges in color from creamy beige to black. Buy it in ready-to-eat cereal or pasta.

Kamut: Another ancient grain, kamut contains 40% more protein than modern hybridized wheat. It has a rich, buttery flavor and can be substitut-

Soy bean products such as tofu,
soy milk, yogurt and cheese,
or soy burgers, bacon and sausages,
are excellent sources of protein.

ed for wheat in most recipes. The whole grain is delicious used in salads or with vegetables. Buy it as pasta or oatmeal-like cereal flakes.

Lupini: Sweet lupin combines with whole wheat flour to create lupini. It stands alone among pastas for its valuable level of beta-carotene and amino acids. Buy this deep brown pasta as spaghetti or in a variety of other shapes.

Healthy Protein-Rich Foods

Protein is necessary for growth and the efficient functioning and repair of all tissues and organs. When asked to name foods containing protein, most people will mention meat, eggs and dairy products. But there are many alternative sources of delicious and easily digestible protein that are not derived from animal sources. Nuts and seeds are an excellent source of protein. While I find them the easiest to digest of all protein-containing foods, I eat them in moderation since they are high in fat. It is worth noting, however, that the fat present in nuts or nut butters is much easier for the body to digest than processed or cooked animal fat.

Soy bean products such as tofu, soy milk, yogurt and cheese, or soy burgers, bacon and sausages, are excellent sources of protein. If possible, substitute any of these soy products for foods containing animal protein. This will

Chinese Cooking Has the Right Answer

Take a tip from Chinese cuisine. Use meat as a garnish. Instead of a steak or half a chicken, slice lean beef or chicken breast paper thin and add it to lightly seasoned steamed vegetables.

improve your health and support the needs of the planet at the same time.

The right combination of whole grains and beans/peas provides your body with the amino acids it needs to manufacture its own complete protein. Soy products are most readily assimilated when combined with non-starchy vegetables or green vegetable salads. As a rule of thumb, fresh salads always assist in the digestion of proteins and starches. People often believe they need more protein than they actually do. In fact, a diet too high in protein can be hard on your body and cause serious problems. Too much protein can overburden your kidneys as they struggle to process the resultant waste products. You could, in fact, end up excreting the calcium you had hoped would benefit your bones and teeth.

Suggested Foods

Years of limiting your fruit and vegetable consumption to several basic choices may have left you with the mistaken impression that vegetarian eating is boring or limited. Nothing could be further from the truth. The following food lists represent much of the natural bounty available for healthy eating. Refer back to it when you are looking for inspiration in your food program.

ALL FRUITS, FRESH AND DRIED

- Apples of all kinds
- Apricots
- Avocados
- Bananas
- Berries of all kinds
- Black Currants
- Breadfruit
- Cactus Fruit
- Cantaloupe
- Cherimoya
- Cherries
- Dates and Date Sugar
- Figs of all kinds
- Grapefruit
- Gooseberries
- Grapes of all kinds
- Guava
- Jack Fruit
- Kiwi
- Kumquats
- Lemons
- Limes
- Loquats
- Mangoes
- Melons of all kinds
- Nectarines
- Olives
- Oranges
- Papaya
- Passion Fruit
- Peaches
- Pears
- Persimmons
- Pineapple
- Plums and Prunes
- Pomegranates
- Raisins
- Sapote or Starapple
- Tangerines
- Tomatoes

ALL VEGETABLES

- Artichokes
- Asparagus
- Bean Sprouts
- Beets and Beet Tops
- Broccoli
- Brussels Sprouts
- Cabbage
- Carrots
- Cauliflower
- Celery
- Chickpeas
- Chives
- Corn
- Cucumbers
- Dandelion Greens
- Eggplant
- Endive
- Garlic
- Jerusalem Artichokes
- Jicama
- Kale
- Kohlrabi
- Leeks
- Lettuce of all kinds
- Mustard Greens
- Okra
- Onions of all kinds
- Parsley
- Peas
- Peppers of all kinds
- Green Bell Pepper
- Potatoes of all kinds
- Radishes
- Rutabagas
- Sauerkraut (raw)
- Spinach
- Sprouts of all kinds
- String Beans
- Summer and Winter Squashes of all kinds
- Turnips
- Turnip Tops
- Watercress
- Yams
- Sweet Potatoes

HERBAL TEAS

Avoid conventional teas which often contain caffeine. Some of my favorite herb teas:

Shave grass tea: *Great for your skin; good for weak kidneys* • Oatstraw tea: *High in silicon; great for nerves; skin; hair and nails* • Peppermint tea: *Keeps your colon healthy; good for stomach trouble and digestion* • Echinacea: *Great for coughing attacks; helps strengthen immune system; helps loosen up mucus in the lungs; great for lymphatic system; a tonic for reproductive system* • Comfrey tea: *Good for anemia; it is said to build blood; helps eliminate mucus from the lungs* • Licorice tea: *Particularly good for the adrenal glands* • Golden Seal: *Great for colds and sore throat; helps strengthen immune system; great for lymphatic system; great for blood circulation*

ALL NUTS AND NUT BUTTERS, NUT "MILKS" AND SEEDS

Use nuts raw and unsalted. Preferably soaked and skinned nuts before consuming.

SWEETENERS

- Barley Malt Syrup
- Blackstrap Molasses
- Brown Rice Syrup
- Date Sugar
- Maple Syrup
- Honey (used sparingly because of its alkalizing properties)

SPICES

- Barbecue Sauce
- Bragg's Liquid Amino
- Cayenne Pepper (add after cooking)
- Jensen's Quick Sip
- Jensen's Vegetable Broth Seasoning
- Kelp and/or Dulse
- Ketchup
- Mustard
- Raw Apple Cider Vinegar
- Natural Condiments with no salt or refined sugar added (may be honey- or juice-sweetened)
- Rice Vinegar

OILS—RAW, UNREFINED, OR COLD-PRESSED

- Avocado
- Canola
- Flax Seed
- Linseed
- Olive
- Peanut
- Safflower
- Sesame
- Sunflower

GRAINS

- Barley
- Brewer's Yeast
- Buckwheat
- Millet
- Oats and Oat Bran
- Rice and Rice Bran
- Rye Grain
- Whole Wheat, Wheat Germ and Wheat Bran

LEGUMES

- Beans and Peas of all kinds
- Bean sprouts
- Carob Powder and Carob Candy
- Hummus
- Peanuts and cashews
- Soybeans and soybean derivatives: Soy milk, cheese, burgers, ice cream, wieners, yogurt, etc.

MISCELLANEOUS

- Fruit-Sweetened Jams
- Vegetarian Burgers: Made from grains and other vegetables
- Vegetarian Bouillon

DAIRY PRODUCTS

Consider substituting soy products for the dairy foods you typically eat. You'll discover that there are many soy products that offer delightful taste without the unhealthy side effects that go along with the consumption of dairy products. If you wish to include raw, unpasteurized milk, yogurt, butter and cheeses, remember they are very concentrated sources of protein and are hard to digest. Use them sparingly.

*Be sure to drink plenty of water
when you eat protein-rich foods.*

Less Is Best

I always recommend if you eat meat, that it be raised organically. It is also in your best interest to buy the leanest available cuts.

The Noble Turkey

Turkeys may have a reputation for being stupid, but they're the smart way to go if you're trying to avoid fat. If poultry is a part of your diet, consider sticking with the white meat of the turkey. One three-ounce portion of turkey breast contains less than one gram of fat. The equivalent boneless, skinless chicken breast has three grams of fat. And watch out for ground chicken. Unless the label says "breast meat," there may be fattier parts of the bird included.

The fat grams shown are for three-ounce cooked portions.
• *turkey breast* — .6 grams
• *chicken breast* — 3 grams
• *beef top round* — 3 grams
• *pork tenderloin* — 4 grams

Be sure to drink plenty of water when you eat protein-rich foods. Water will help your body digest and assimilate these foods with greater efficiency. Water also flushes out the waste products of protein digestion, such as uric acid, which can accumulate over time and cause unwelcome side effects. Animal products are notorious for leaving toxic waste products in the system. Vegetarian protein does not impact the system in such a negative way.

Availability of Fresh Fruits/Vegetables

Another factor which discourages many people from adopting a vegetarian diet is the modest selection of fresh produce. Prices are high and choices quite limited in many places, especially during the winter months. Here in Los Angeles, there is an abundant selection of locally grown fresh produce at good prices. The climate in L.A. is warm year-round, so it is relatively easy for me to maintain my strict regimen. Each of us has the opportunity to choose a lifestyle that supports our health needs. This book is designed to make you more aware of food combinations and dietary possibilities. As I have said before, experiment and find out what works best for you.

One should eat to live,
not live to eat.

Marcus Tullius Cicero (106 BC - 43 BC)

Roman orator, statesman and philosopher

The Aspartame Debate

Aspartame, the artificial sweetener sold as NutraSweet, is still the subject of considerable debate in scientific communities. Some studies report that it increases appetite. Others contradict this finding. There are anecdotal data that suggest aspartame was responsible for causing headaches and grand-mal seizures. Yet many mothers have offered it to their children for years without incident. Generally, artificial sweeteners are of greater benefit to the corporations that manufacture them than they are to the consumers who use them.

The best way to use proteins is with raw or nearly raw vegetables. The enzymes in the vegetables help the body assimilate the protein. Vegetable fiber helps bulk up the concentrated proteins which also assists the digestive process. Your optimal diet should contain 75% or more of raw food. Cooked foods should be lightly steamed or baked at low heat. High heat destroys food value and the live elements in foodstuffs.

Foods to Avoid

The following foods take too long to digest, are too concentrated, and unless organic, may contain toxic substances:

• *Seafood*
   Any pickled, smoked or processed Seafoods
• *Red Meat*
   Veal, Beef, Pork or Liver Products
• *Poultry*
   Chicken, Turkey (especially the skin)
• *Refined White Flour Products*
   Bread, Cakes, Cookies, Waffles, Pancakes, Enchiladas, Pizza Crust, Creamy Soups, Tacos, Macaroni, Spaghetti, Crackers, Gravies, Noodles, etc. (The refining process removes the important vitamins and minerals.)
• *White Sugar Products*
   Sodas, Syrups, Juices, Jellies, Jams, Cakes, Candies, Cookies, Pies, etc.
• *Pasteurized Dairy Products*
   Milk, Cream Cheese, Ice Cream
• *Cocoa and Chocolate*
• *Conventional Tea and Coffee*

So many fruits and vegetables are preserved by waxing, which can be toxic. Remember to peel the fruit or vegetable to remove the wax coating, especially apples and cucumbers.

Commercial varieties contain caffeine; exceptions include most herbal teas and decaffeinated coffees.

- *Cigarettes and other Tobacco Products*
- *Alcohol*
  Liquors, beer and wine
- *Salt*
- *Ascorbic Acid*
- *Fried Foods*
  Potato Chips, Fried Rice, French Fries, Fried Pies, Donuts, etc.
- *Preservatives and Additives*
  These are found virtually everywhere in conventional oils, bakery goods, fats, cereals, desserts, canned foods and many prepared foods. (Read labels carefully. Watch out for sodium dioxide, sodium benzoate, or sulfur dioxide in fruit juices and dried fruits. MSG, BHT, BHA, nitrates and nitrites and cream of tartar are all damaging to your body.)
- *Roasted and Salted Nuts*
  These foods form acid in your system.
- *Commercial Seasonings*
  Ketchup, mustard, horseradish, relishes, pickles, bottled sauces and dressings contain preservatives, sugar and salt.
- *Commercial Waxed Produce*
  So many fruits and vegetables are preserved by waxing, which can be toxic. Remember to peel the fruit or vegetable to remove the wax coating, especially apples and cucumbers.

Living Well Really Is the Best Revenge!

Many manufacturers have gotten wise to the fact that Americans are paying more attention to their health. But don't assume these manufacturers are out to help you. For example, "natural" has yet to be defined by the FDA. Many "natural" products are crammed with fats, sugars and preservatives. Watch out for "light" and "lite" as well.

- *Saturated Fats, Hydrogenated Oils*
  These foods are high in saturated acids and often contain rancid factors. Avoid butter, cream, ice cream, whole milk cheeses, margarines, hardened shortenings (Crisco, etc.), non-dairy creamers, mayonnaise, cottonseed oil,

Some of the strongest, most intelligent, beautiful and long-lived animals are not meat eaters. We are fortunate to share the planet with many vegetarian species: small animals like rabbits and squirrels, and larger animals like camels, deer, oxen, sheep, cows, goats, horses, elephants, apes and monkeys!

soy oil, coconut oil, lard, salted peanut butter, and all hydrogenated oils.
- *Salted Foods*
- *Commercial Seasonings and Dressings*
  Canned sauerkraut, olives, pretzels, potato and corn chips, crackers, commercial dry cereals, breads and cakes, commercially prepared Chinese foods, smoked meats (including fish and poultry), canned soups and other canned foods, some frozen foods.
- *Miscellaneous*
  Aspirin, sleeping pills, pain killers, milk of magnesia, commercial laxatives, sprouted or green-tinged potatoes.

A Little Food for (Vegetarian) Thought

How do other species obtain their protein? Some of the strongest, most intelligent, beautiful and long-lived animals are not meat eaters. We are fortunate to share the planet with many vegetarian species: small animals like rabbits and squirrels, and larger animals like camels, deer, oxen, sheep, cows, goats, horses, elephants, apes and monkeys! Observed in their natural habitats, these species graze, forage or gather their protein from the vegetable-rich environs in which they dwell. Meat-eating animals, on the other hand, are known to be scavengers. They are killers of other species and contrary to our impressions of their strength, they are the weakest and most dependent when born. This includes housecats, leopards, tigers, lions, rats and hyenas.

Vegetarianism is not a modern invention. We have evidence that there were whole communities that avoided animal foods even in ancient times. Pythagoras, the Greek philosopher, advocated millet and sesame seeds as the best source of protein. If you become a vegetarian, you'll be joining such historical luminaries as Shelley, Shaw, Ovid, Plato, Socrates, Einstein, Darwin, da Vinci, Wagner, Aristotle, Plutarch, Alexander the Great, Newton, Tolstoy, Emerson, Lord Buddha, Krishna, Mahatma Ghandi, Albert Schweitzer and Voltaire, to name only a few. Dave Scott, the only man to win the Ironman Triathlon more than twice, is a vegetarian.

While few meat and potato fans are likely to convert to complete vegetarianism overnight, the first step on the path to an environmentally sound diet is easy. One day a week, substitute a vegetarian main course for one containing meat. If you have trouble giving up meat, try eating less at each sitting. Eat more salads, vegetables, grains and bean dishes instead. Perhaps you're ready to cut your meat consumption by half. You'll be rewarded with immediate health benefits. There are plenty of vegetarian cookbooks available, and most restaurants have meatless meals on their menus. Some people

The natural world provides us with many clues about healthful living if we take the time to examine them.

choose to give up red meat but continue to eat fish and poultry. Others give up all animal products, including eggs and dairy products. I have come to actually prefer a diet of mostly fruits and nuts, with some vegetables and occasional grains and beans.

As you make decisions about what to include in your diet, consider the following: The human digestive system most resembles that of other plant- and fruit-eating primates. Like other primates, man's intestinal tract, at six times his body length, is designed to digest well-chewed vegetables, grains and fruits. Our twelve molar teeth are adapted to grinding, the better to chew our foods. The pH value of our saliva closely resembles that of other vegetarian primates.

By contrast, the intestinal tract of a carnivore is relatively short and only three times the length of its body. This abbreviated digestive path allows for rapid expulsion of the potentially toxic waste products typically found in flesh. It is also worth noting that the large canine teeth of most carnivores are adapted to tearing rather than chewing food. The natural world provides us with many clues about healthful living if we take the time to examine them.

Avoid Pesticides, Buy Organically Grown Foods!

Commercial agriculture in this country is all about producing large crops for profitable distribution. In our rush to eradicate garden pests and plant diseases, we spray our food supply with cancer-causing pesticides. Common products like malathion, benomyl and diazinon are available to home gardeners as well as the giants of commercial agriculture now farming much of our land. Many pesticides approved for use by the Environmental Protection Agency (EPA) were registered long before extensive research linked these chemicals to cancer and other diseases. Now the EPA has established that over 60% of all herbicides, over 90% of all fungicides, and over 30% of all insecticides are carcinogenic. No pesticide is 100% safe. The bottom line is that the highly poisonous pesticides designed to kill living organisms are also harmful to human beings. In addition to cancer, pesticides are implicated in birth defects, nerve damage and genetic mutation.

But there is good news. From the roadside stand to the produce section of your local supermarket to mail-order suppliers, organic produce is becoming increasingly available. The produce should carry a "certified organic" label listing the certifying organization. Many towns and cities have farmer's markets where growers of organic fruits and vegetables will be happy to talk to you about their commitment to growing pesticide-free produce. Mail-order delivery of organic produce may also be available in your area. Ask your local

*Be sure to wash your veggies and fruit
before eating, and always use a vegetable brush
on potatoes if you plan to eat the skin.*

health food store about local distributors. In addition, the National Organic Directory, which lists distributors of organic produce, can be ordered by calling the community Alliance of Family Farmers at (800) 952-3832. The cost of the directory is $34.95 plus shipping and handling. Remember, organic produce cannot be expected to last as long as those commercially grown fruits and vegetables bred and treated to have an extended shelf life.

Finally, if you are unable to find organically grown produce, or unwilling to pay the higher cost, be sure to wash your veggies and fruit before eating, and always use a vegetable brush on potatoes if you plan to eat the skin.

For questions about pesticides, call the EPA-sponsored National Pesticide Telecommunications Network at (800) 858-7378.

Non-toxic Solutions

Planting your own organic vegetables can be easier than you think. Tomatoes can be raised in pots on high-rise balconies! If you decide to try a modest backyard garden, consider these tips:

Don't Bug Me!

This may not work in mosquito-infested woods, but it will keep the biting pests away when you're on a picnic in the park.

Combine 2 cups witch hazel with 1½ teaspoons oil of citronella and 1 tablespoon apple cider vinegar. Pour into spritzer and shake vigorously. Apply to entire body when needed. Safe for children too!

• Choose seeds and plants that are likely to thrive in your climate.
• Your local nursery has easy-to-use kits that enable you to test your soil to find out how to feed it properly.
• Overplant! Your garden will never be a total loss.
• Learn about companion planting. Particular groupings of plants and herbs have been found to support each other's healthy growth. Basil, coriander and thyme are among the fragrant herbs that offer protection against common garden pests.
• Make your own non-toxic pesticide. Sprinkle a mixture of baking soda, garlic juice and hot pepper on the problem area.

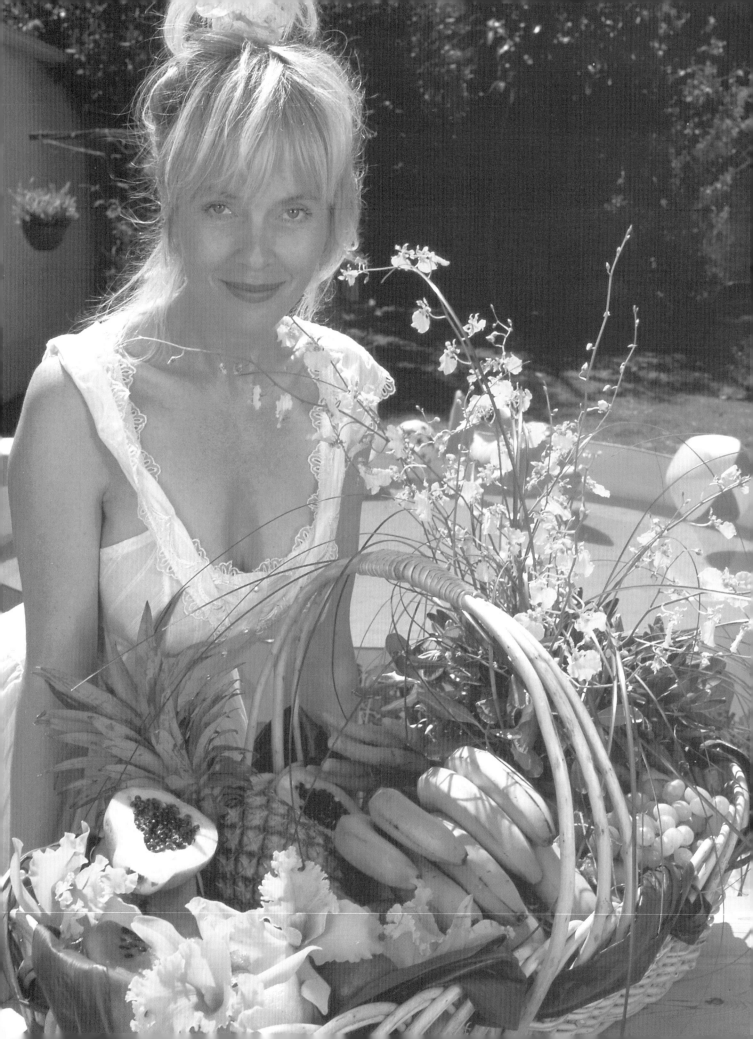

CHAPTER TWO

Food Combining

The digestive process breaks down complex foodstuffs for utilization by the body. We may experience food as "good or bad," sweet or sour, fattening or not. But our digestive systems experience proteins, carbohydrates, sugars or fats as specific chemical compounds, each requiring a different type of digestive secretion. When we mix our foods without regard to their varying metabolic needs, digestion is less efficient.

The secret to healthy metabolism is successful food combining. The basic premise is this: When foods are improperly combined, the rapid metabolism of food into vital body-building nutrients is slowed down. Our bodies are not designed to absorb and assimilate too many different types of foods at one sitting. Let's say you eat a big, juicy steak with a baked potato and all the trimmings. First, your digestive system must produce several secretions to assimilate your dinner. Then, these incompatible digestive juices mix with the contents of your stomach, trying to begin digestion. But your metabolic process is already slowed down, hopelessly at odds with itself. The steak begins to decompose and the potato ferments before digestion can be completed. The result is the uncomfortable feeling of gas and bloating with which we're all familiar. As you loosen your belt a notch, and vow never to overeat again, your brain sends a signal to your pancreas to secrete more digestive juices. This causes the pancreas to go into overdrive. Although your digestive system is on red alert, it is functioning at a severely compromised

I am convinced digestion
is the great secret of life.

Sydney Smith (1771 - 1845) English clergyman, essayist and wit

level. It can actually take over thirty-six hours to complete this process and rid the body of resulting wastes. By now, you have spent the better part of a day feeling sluggish and wishing you could slip into bed for a nap. Returning to my original analogy of efficient performance, it is easy to see that appropriate food combinations are absolutely crucial for peak metabolic efficiency.

Let's look at an unsuccessful vegetarian food combination. How about an apple cut up with walnuts and raisins. Sounds healthy enough. But in this case the combination of protein (walnuts) and sugar (apples and raisins) will result in the decomposition of the walnuts and the fermentation of the raisins. Again, you are left feeling bloated. If a carbohydrate and sugar are eaten together, both the carbohydrate and the sugar ferment, leaving you with the same uncomfortable, gassy sensation.

These unsuccessful food combinations deplete the body's resources and prevent it from performing other vital functions such as burning fat and supplying energy. In addition, healthy cell structure cannot be built from decomposed and fermented components, so as the body expends valuable energy to overcome its digestive obstacles, the food offers diminished nutritive value and is less useful as fuel. As a result of allowing undigested or partially digested food particles through our systems, waste products are produced, frequently yielding harmful toxins. These toxins place a great strain on our cells, the tissues of our bodies, and our organs of elimination. That is why we experience symptoms like gas, bloating and sour stomach.

Our bodies are extraordinarily forgiving, but that can be the bad news as well as the good. The signs of poor health can be subtle. Many of us simply get used to feeling a little "off." Too frequently we assume that exhaustion comes with the territory of our busy lives. But food combining has provided many with the key to renewed energy.

Three Basic Types of Food

In examining the variables of proper food combining, we break down all foods into three fundamental areas:
• *Concentrated* (proteins and carbohydrates)
• *Low concentration, high water content* (fruits and vegetables)
• *Fats*
• Proteins, because of their high concentration, require the most time and energy to digest and assimilate—usually two to six hours. At two to four hours, carbohydrates take just a little less time. Fruits are the least concentrated foods and require only one hour to assimilate.
• All fruits—with the exception of bananas, dried fruit and avocados—pass

Fruit eaten at the end of a meal
is forced to wait its digestive turn and
ferments in the stomach and intestine.
Fruit eaten separately or before a meal is
provided with clear digestive passage.

directly through the stomach and digest in the intestines. Fruit eaten at the end of a meal is forced to wait its digestive turn and ferments in the stomach and intestine. Fruit eaten separately or before a meal is provided with clear digestive passage. Fats and oils require little stomach activity and usually inhibit the flow of hydrochloric acid to the stomach. When fats are consumed along with proteins, which require the activity of stomach juices, digestion is greatly slowed down, if not completely stopped. This alone is the cause of much stomach distress.

Awakening to a New System

Before I learned about food combining, I sometimes felt poorly even though I was eating healthy food. I experienced indigestion or a burning sensation, and frequently felt bloated. I even had headaches. I now realize this was due to lumping all kinds of food together in the same meal. As long as I was eating healthy foods, I thought my stomach would tolerate any mixture I wanted to eat. However, I learned from my many mistakes. Since mastering the science of food combining, I have experienced few digestive problems.

Using the food combinations nature intended places a minimal load on the digestive organs, thereby preserving their health and vigor over a lifetime. Foods can be easily and properly assimilated and waste products eliminated resulting in the pure bloodstream which is essential to maintenance of a strong, vital body.

Even within the confines of a conventional American diet, gastrointestinal complaints could be dramatically reduced through successful food combining. Many smart, educated people, even medical doctors, eat all kinds of foods that do not combine well. When they get indigestion, they take antacids to rid themselves of the problem. In fact, this is such a common way to deal with digestive problems, many take their doses as a matter of course, and don't regard these "remedies" as medication.

Prevention!

Why not prevent the problem from occurring in the first place? Why fill your sensitive stomach with foods that fight each other for digestive attention? Why cause your digestive system to work overtime and then cure the crisis by reaching into the medicine cabinet?

The good news is that it is easy to avoid these problems without sacrificing great tasting meals. By applying a knowledge of food combining, we can eat any number of foods, in an almost infinite variety.

Safeguard the health of both body and soul.

Cleobulus

Easy Rules of Food Combination

- First and foremost, never overeat any food.
- Do not eat fruit with any other food. Fruit is best eaten alone or at least fifteen minutes before the main course begins. Fruit washes and cleanses the digestive system and makes it capable of better absorbing other nutrients.
- Eat melon alone or leave it alone . . . How easy to remember!
- Do not eat too many varieties of foods at any one meal.
- Always eat a leafy green salad with any food containing protein, carbohydrate or fat.
- Do not combine starches with sugars.
- Do not combine starches with animal protein.
- Never eat fruit as a dessert. This is a sure way to get indigestion and interfere with the food value of the meal you just ate. (Exception: Papaya)
- Tomatoes may be eaten with non-starchy vegetables and protein.
- Avocado is best with acid or sub-acid fruit or green vegetables.
- Combine vegetables with either starches or animal protein. Do not combine these three different types of foods at one sitting.
- Seeds are fine accompaniments to all types of food. Soak them for several hours to bring out flavor and to make them easier to digest.
- Use fresh, unprocessed whole foods, if available. Use very few refined, frozen and canned foods.
- When possible, eat foods that have been organically grown.

For easy digestion, it is also important to chew your food until it liquifies. The digestive process is also slowed down by spices, vinegar, tobacco, alcohol, soft drinks, tea, coffee and iced drinks you may consume along with your meal.

Salads Aid Digestion

If you eat a fatty protein such as a steak, a mixed vegetable salad will help offset the inhibiting effect upon your digestion. Dairy products are also difficult to digest. If they are eaten, they should be served with a salad. Proteins, meats and carbohydrates (starches) should also be consumed with a salad or steamed vegetables for optimum digestion.

Raw tomatoes are an acidic fruit, but they enter the digestive tract in an extremely alkaline form, thus helping to neutralize acid buildup in the system. Cooked tomatoes, however, are extremely acid-forming and damaging to the internal organs. If you must have spaghetti sauce on your pasta, make sure you eat a big, green salad alongside.

Food combining is an important tool in the battle against excess weight. The answer to a weight problem is not in dieting, but in healthy food choices and thoughtful food combining and consistent exercise.

Carbohydrates and Sugars

Bread is easier to digest and forms less mucus in your body when toasted. I usually choose a sprouted grain bread. I like to put organically grown bananas and fruit-sweetened jam on no-salt whole grain bread. I know that mixing sugary fruit and starchy bread is not a recommended food combination, but it is a vast improvement on "the white flour and candy diet" that continues to tempt me occasionally. Even healthy starches and fruit sugars are not compatible. This combination can lead to fermentation and a sour stomach and can generate alcohols and aldehydes which tend to destroy red corpuscles. Starchy foods require the action of the starch-splitting enzyme ptyalin while sugars do not. If sugar is eaten along with starchy foods, ptyalin will not be present in the saliva. Consequently, when the starchy food enters the intestinal tract, it will not be properly prepared for digestion in the stomach.

Excess Weight and Fatigue

Food combining is an important tool in the battle against excess weight. Without food combining, the energy that should be available to break down and eliminate excess fat is instead put to use in the digestive system. There is not enough energy at the body's disposal to carry out the functions of digestion and elimination of unneeded fat, resulting inevitably in excess weight. The burden put on the digestive processes in this scenario must be reversed. When you remove excess weight, you enhance your chances to live free of debilitating ailments.

A ten-year study at the New York Obesity Research Center at Rockefeller University shows that the body will go to great lengths to maintain the weight it had at the beginning of any calorie restricted diet. The results of the study indicate that the body suddenly deprived of calories will slow its own metabolism by reducing the number of calories needed for basic body functions like breathing, blood circulation and digestion. At the same time, muscle efficiency is increased so that fewer calories are burned during exercise.

The diet industry in this country has grown fat on the naive hopes of millions of Americans. The C. Everett Koop Foundation reports that the United States spends more than $400 billion annually in health costs related to obesity. I watched with horror as a friend of mine dropped sixty-five pounds on a liquid diet and gained it all back with interest in less than a year. The answer to a weight problem is not in dieting, but in healthy food choices and thoughtful food combining and consistent exercise. All of us have known someone who appears to eat with abandon and never gains weight. In addition to restraining ourselves from thinking evil thoughts

The only diet that works is the diet that changes the way you eat for a lifetime.

about them, we are well advised to pay attention to their lifestyle. While they may say they eat like stevedores, it is more likely that they work out like longshoremen. Scientists tell us what many of us know instinctively. The only diet that works is the diet that changes the way you eat for a lifetime.

Examples of Healthy Food Combinations

Fruit Smoothies: All different kinds of fruits can be used, even frozen fruits, with seeds if desired. Sunflower seeds and sesame are two of the best. See the recipe chapter for some ideas.

Fruit Plates/Salads: Add some lettuce and celery to your fruit salad plate.

Vegetable Salad: Raw vegetable combinations make tasty vegetable salads. You can also add some steamed vegetables. Combine the mixture with whole raw nuts and seeds to include protein. If you want to add other vegetarian protein, there are many tofu products from which to choose. If you eat animal protein, select lean cuts of organically grown beef, chicken or turkey, eggs, milk products or fish from clean waters to embellish your salad. Organically grown animal products have no hormones or antibiotics in them.

Energy Soup: Liquefy a variety of raw vegetables in your blender, perhaps with a little lemon juice. Especially good are spinach, lettuce, cucumber, tomato, sprouts, celery and avocado.

Energy Dip: Even a whole vegetable salad can be puréed with ripe avocado in the blender to make a dip.

Mixed Steamed Vegetable Plate: Eat vegetables alone, with starches (brown rice, baked potato, vegetarian burger) or with animal proteins. Tofu, prepared in a variety of ways, is an excellent source of vegetarian protein. Non-vegetarians can enjoy baked and broiled fish, fowl, beef and cheeses with their steamed vegetables. Never eat starches and animal proteins with your vegetarian plate at any one meal. Choose one or the other.

Veggie Stews: Combine your favorite vegetables, potatoes, grains, beans, etc. and perhaps have a slice of bread alongside.

Protein-Veggie Stews: Never eat starches and proteins together, but you may

Both grains and legumes contain more nutritional value for the human body once they have been sprouted.

want to cook non-starchy vegetables with animal proteins or eat a slice of cheese with steamed vegetables.

Spaghetti: Whole wheat pasta, enhanced for color and flavor through the use of vegetables in preparation, is widely available. The addition of steamed or sautéed vegetables makes a gourmet meal. Use raw salsa or fresh tomato sauce to spice up this dish.

Recommended Salad Ingredients

Leafy Greens: All lettuces, spinach, cabbage, sprouts, beet tops, swiss chard, parsley, among others.

Summer Squash: Varieties like zucchini and crookneck.

Roots: Beets, jicama, carrots.

Other: Cucumber, tomato, green pepper, cauliflower, broccoli, okra, string beans, peas, kohlrabi, among others.

Recommended Vegetables for Steaming and Baking

Choose your seasonal favorites and those which are locally available: hard squashes, potatoes, yams and other tubers, sweet corn, kohlrabi, parsnips, Brussels sprouts, cabbage, pumpkin, collard greens, swiss chard, beets, carrots, kale, dandelion, peas, string beans and eggplant.

Recommended Carbohydrates

Alkaline Carbos: Bananas, dates, figs, avocados, potatoes, yams, sweet potatoes, sweet corn, dried fruits, carob, coconut and chestnuts.

Acid Starches/Carbos: All grains and their products, all dried beans and peas. Both grains and legumes contain more nutritional value for the human body once they have been sprouted.

Fresh Fruits: Sweet oranges, grapefruit, pineapple, tangerines, sweet apples, pears, plums, nectarines, peaches, apricots, all berries, cherries, all melons, grapes, mangoes, cheremoyas, guavas, persimmons, among others.

Keep your eyes open for hidden fats
in pre-packaged products like crackers.
They are frequently made with unhealthy
hydrogenated oils.

Recommended Protein

Nuts: Almonds, cashews, filberts, macadamias, walnuts, pecans, pignolias, pistachios.
Seeds: Sunflower seeds, pumpkin seeds, sesame seeds.

Some Legumes: Including peanuts, soybeans, lentils. To gain the maximum nutritional value from legumes, eat them in their sprouted form. Sprouted soybeans are delicious in salads.
Milk: From nuts, seeds or soybeans.

Goat's Milk: Raw and unpasteurized, especially for infants and children.

All nuts, including peanuts, are best eaten raw.
While all nuts and seeds contain a lot of protein, they are very rich in fat and should be eaten sparingly. They are a valuable protein source in the winter time, but in hotter weather I eat them only rarely.

Use the following sources of animal protein in moderation.
Eggs: Preferably prepared without butter or margarine.

Cheese: Soft, unsalted cheeses or unsalted Italian Ricotta are best.

Animal Flesh: Beef, pork, fowl, seafood.

Cow's Milk and Milk Products: Raw, unpasteurized dairy products are much better for you than pasteurized products.

Recommended Fats
Raw avocado, cold-pressed or unrefined olive and flax seed oils, and raw, unpasteurized butter used sparingly. Keep your eyes open for hidden fats in pre-packaged products like crackers. They are frequently made with unhealthy hydrogenated oils.

A Word of Encouragement
When I first learned the rules of healthy food combining, I found the process somewhat confusing. It was new territory to me, but I stuck with it because I wanted to see if it would benefit my day-to-day living. I focused a lot of time and energy on the subject. However, I began to observe very pos-

*Although I recommend that fruit
should never be consumed at the end of a meal,
papaya is the exception to the rule.
Papaya enzymes act as a natural aid to digestion.*

itive health benefits right away so I persisted. The first week was the hardest, but the second week was slightly easier. After about six weeks, it became totally automatic to combine my foods correctly.

I have developed a series of menus to help anyone make a successful transition to healthier eating. These are not meant to be followed religiously,

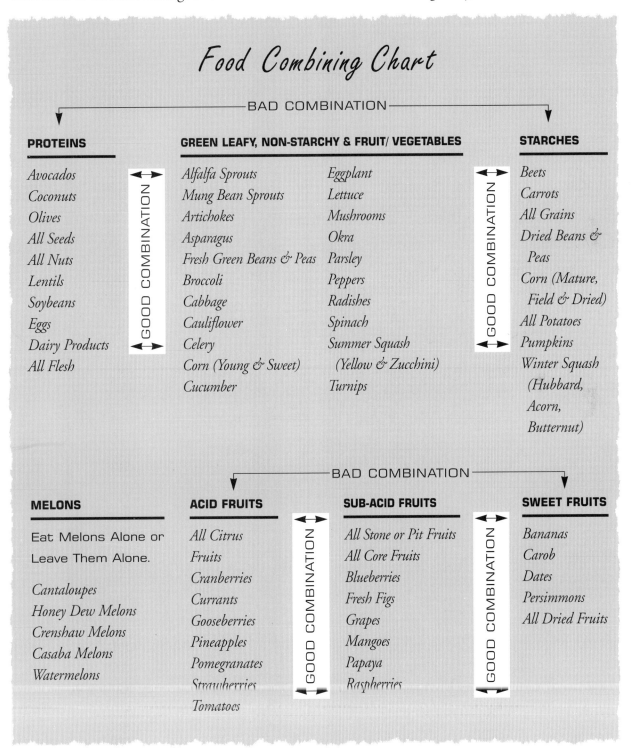

Food Combining Chart

BAD COMBINATION

PROTEINS

Avocados
Coconuts
Olives
All Seeds
All Nuts
Lentils
Soybeans
Eggs
Dairy Products
All Flesh

GOOD COMBINATION

GREEN LEAFY, NON-STARCHY & FRUIT/ VEGETABLES

Alfalfa Sprouts	Eggplant
Mung Bean Sprouts	Lettuce
Artichokes	Mushrooms
Asparagus	Okra
Fresh Green Beans & Peas	Parsley
Broccoli	Peppers
Cabbage	Radishes
Cauliflower	Spinach
Celery	Summer Squash
Corn (Young & Sweet)	(Yellow & Zucchini)
Cucumber	Turnips

GOOD COMBINATION

STARCHES

Beets
Carrots
All Grains
Dried Beans &
    Peas
Corn (Mature,
    Field & Dried)
All Potatoes
Pumpkins
Winter Squash
    (Hubbard,
    Acorn,
    Butternut)

BAD COMBINATION

MELONS

Eat Melons Alone or
Leave Them Alone.

Cantaloupes
Honey Dew Melons
Crenshaw Melons
Casaba Melons
Watermelons

ACID FRUITS

All Citrus
Fruits
Cranberries
Currants
Gooseberries
Pineapples
Pomegranates
Strawberries
Tomatoes

GOOD COMBINATION

SUB-ACID FRUITS

All Stone or Pit Fruits
All Core Fruits
Blueberries
Fresh Figs
Grapes
Mangoes
Papaya
Raspberries

GOOD COMBINATION

SWEET FRUITS

Bananas
Carob
Dates
Persimmons
All Dried Fruits

Menus

Recipes for some menu items can be found in Chapter Four, "Recipes." Remember, you do not have to eat every menu item. Beverages consumed with meals should be sipped in moderation.

THE BEGINNER'S DIET

Beginner profile: This person eats fruits, vegetables, seeds, nuts, grains, beans, meat and dairy products. She avoids hydrogenated oils, and is checking possible food purchases for preservatives, chemicals, refined sugar and salt. Beginner's menus provide many healthy, delicious foods but do not attempt to adhere strictly to the rules of food combining.

Monday
- *breakfast:* fruit juice, soaked peaches, oatmeal, eggs (not fried)
- *lunch:* peppermint tea, cottage cheese and strawberries, chicken salad
- *dinner:* fresh vegetable juice, roast leg of lamb with mashed potatoes and peas, vegetable salad, fresh papaya with a splash of lime. (Although I recommend that fruit should never be consumed at the end of a meal, papaya is the exception to the rule. Papaya enzymes act as a natural aid to digestion. You can even purchase papaya enzyme tablets at your health food store.)

Tuesday
- *breakfast:* Oatstraw tea, fresh pineapple juice, sliced pears, fruit-sweetened corn flakes with soy milk or low-fat milk, rye crackers with raw cheese
- *lunch:* fruit juice, buckwheat pancakes with strawberries and a touch of cream
- *dinner:* fresh carrot juice, steamed fish with lemon, steamed spinach, baby red potatoes, mixed green salad

Wednesday
- *breakfast:* shave grass tea, fresh grapefruit juice, soaked prunes, quinoa cereal with rice milk and maple syrup
- *lunch:* fresh vegetable juice, omelet with mushrooms, bell peppers and tomatoes, steamed beets with chopped onions and celery
- *dinner:* soy milk, vegetarian burger with all the trimmings (sautéed onions, relish, ketchup and mustard)

Thursday
- *breakfast:* echinacea tea, yogurt with fresh pineapple, cornmeal cereal with rice milk
- *lunch:* roasted turkey and potatoes, sautéed kale and cabbage, "milkshake" of fresh apple/celery juice blended with blanched almonds (delicious!)
- *dinner:* fresh carrot/celery juice, vegetable stew with french or sourdough bread, coleslaw

Friday
- *breakfast:* fresh apple juice, golden seal tea, soaked apricots with nut milk, sliced peaches
- *lunch:* soy milk, whole grain pancakes with maple syrup, cottage cheese with diced bell peppers and

chopped parsley
- *dinner:* fresh carrot/zucchini juice, Chinese prepared vegetables, bok choy/cucumber salad

Saturday
- *breakfast:* fresh orange juice, licorice tea, sliced nectarines with cream, millet cereal with soy milk and maple syrup
- *lunch:* carrot juice, sliced oranges and bananas, Rye-Crisp with soy or low-fat cheese and chopped green onion
- *dinner:* soy or low-fat milk, broiled lean steak with grilled leeks and summer squash, mixed green salad with sun dried tomatoes

Sunday
- *breakfast:* flax seed tea, fresh figs, muesli with banana and dates, low-fat milk, soft- or hard-boiled egg
- *lunch:* fresh carrot/cucumber/beet juice, tofu wieners on a bun or with mashed potatoes, garnish of raw or grilled onions and pickles, ketchup, mustard
- *dinner:* smoothie (any fruit combo), grilled or roasted chicken (no skin!), peas and green beans (raw or steamed), mixed green salad

THE INTERMEDIATE DIET

Intermediate profile: This person eats fruit, vegetables, seeds, nuts, grains and beans. While she continues to use some dairy foods, there are minimal animal products in her diet. She does not use hydrogenated oils, and has made a commitment to avoid unhealthful chemical additives and preservatives in her food choices. She has found healthy alternatives to refined salt, sugar and flour products.

Monday
- *breakfast:* fresh fruit juice, melon, nut butter with celery sticks
- *lunch:* fresh vegetable juice, coleslaw, veggie or soy burger with all the trimmings (see Beginner's Diet)
- *dinner:* herbal tea, steamed or marinated beets, vegetable stew

Tuesday
- *breakfast:* fresh fruit juice, grapes, jicama sticks, nut butter
- *lunch:* fresh vegetable juice, grated carrots and beets, steamed asparagus, red skin potatoes
- *dinner:* herbal tea, vegetarian chili, lettuce, alfalfa sprout and avocado salad

Wednesday
- *breakfast:* fresh fruit juice, strawberries and bananas
- *lunch:* fresh vegetable juice, green salad with hummus, corn bread
- *dinner:* herbal tea, mixed green salad, soy cheese pizza with sautéed vegetable topping (including onion, garlic, bell peppers, Japanese eggplant, yellow squash)

Thursday
- *breakfast:* herbal tea, banana, papaya, pineapple and sesame seed smoothie
- *lunch:* fresh vegetable juice, corn chips with salsa and guacamole
- *dinner:* fresh apple/carrot juice, vegetable stick salad, corn on the cob, soy wiener with all the trimmings, a handful of baked potato chips

Friday
- *breakfast:* apple, raspberry and banana smoothie, dried figs
- *lunch:* fresh vegetable juice, herbal tea, cucumber, lettuce, tomato and avocado with soy mayonnaise on sprouted grain toast (or sprinkle dulse, kelp or vegetable seasoning on toast and enjoy your salad on the side)
- *dinner:* soy milk, barley vegetable soup, sourdough bread with raw butter or seasoned olive oil, mixed green and alfalfa sprout salad

Saturday
- *breakfast:* apple, peach and banana smoothie, tangerines, yogurt
- *lunch:* sliced tomato with red onions and seasoned olive oil, baked red skin potatoes split open and topped with steamed, sliced broccoli (pile a little of the tomato/onion mixture on top as well—it's delicious!)
- *dinner:* fresh carrot/beet juice, herbal tea, stew of peas, lentils and various vegetables (soy wieners or bacon can be added for variety), dinner rolls

Sunday
- *breakfast:* fresh orange/strawberry juice, bananas, soy yogurt or low-fat macadamia nut ice cream
- *lunch:* herbal tea, cottage cheese with pineapple chunks, corn meal pancakes with maple syrup
- *dinner:* fresh carrot juice, nut milk, sautéed vegetables with tofu chunks and brown rice, tomato, avocado, green onion, celery and bell pepper salad topped with fresh grated garlic

THE ADVANCED DIET

Advanced profile: This person eats fruit, vegetables, seeds and nuts. She has made the decision to avoid all animal products, substituting rice, soy or nut milks for dairy products. Her consumption of commercially prepared food products is minimal.

Monday
- *breakfast:* fresh orange juice, grapes and bananas, almond milk
- *lunch:* fresh carrot/apple juice, vegetable salad with slivered almonds
- *dinner:* fresh carrot/cucumber juice, celery sticks with nut butter, steamed cauliflower and yellow squash

Tuesday
- *breakfast:* fresh apple juice, melon, sesame/sunflower seed milk
- *lunch:* fresh carrot/zucchini juice, steamed string beans, sautéed cabbage and leeks, baked potatoes, jicama sticks
- *dinner:* carrot/celery juice, vegetable salad with mixed sprouts and avocado, handful of pecans

Wednesday
- *breakfast:* fresh pineapple juice, soaked apricots with banana and shredded coconut
- *lunch:* fresh carrot/beet juice, mixed green salad with avocado, handful of filberts
- *dinner:* carrot juice, steamed broccoli and artichoke, coleslaw

Thursday
- *breakfast:* fresh apple/strawberry juice, coconut milk, dates and bananas
- *lunch:* fresh carrot juice, Raw Energy Soup, handful of walnuts
- *dinner:* fresh carrot/beet/cucumber juice, steamed peas, carrots and white potatoes, sliced tomato and avocado with dulse powder

Friday
- *breakfast:* apple, peach and banana smoothie, dried figs, cashew nut milk
- *lunch:* fresh carrot/zucchini juice, vegetable stick salad, handful of macadamia nuts
- *dinner:* carrot juice, sautéed kale with onion and garlic, baked yams

Saturday
- *breakfast:* apple, raspberry and banana smoothie, pineapple slices, almond milk
- *lunch:* fresh carrot/beet/cucumber juice, mixed green salad with tomato and avocado, handful of pumpkin seeds
- *dinner:* fresh carrot/apple/zucchini juice, mashed potatoes and cauliflower, grated beets

Sunday
- *breakfast:* fresh orange juice, banana, baked apples sprinkled with nuts
- *lunch:* fresh apple/celery juice blended with blanched almonds, mixed sprout salad with sliced avocado
- *dinner:* fresh carrot/beet juice, vegetable stew, guacamole with celery sticks

*Let correct food combining be one of the factors
that enables you to have a more productive,
enjoyable and abundant life.*

but are merely examples of the different levels. Remember, this is not about deprivation. It is about making positive changes in your life. By providing you with three week-long eating plans, I hope to jump start your commitment to improved health. Don't hesitate to start with the beginner's plan, and stay at each level for as many weeks as you like. Try preparing meals from each of the levels, and mix and match. The important thing is that you will be taking steps to turn your body into the efficient, energetic performer it is designed to be.

Do I "fall off the wagon" on occasion? Absolutely! But I have worked with this system for many years now and when my diet is unhealthy I feel it almost immediately. That, in turn, sends me back to a diet free of the discomfort caused by gas, bloat, indigestion or acid stomach. When I am following the food program that is right for me, I never experience headaches or that "heavy" feeling after a meal. And maybe most important of all, I have the energy and vitality to keep up with the rigorous needs of my young child. The transition has definitely been worth the initial effort! Let correct food combining be one of the factors that enables you to have a more productive, enjoyable and abundant life.

Cooking Tips

- *Use stainless steel cook pots and utensils.*
- *Avoid aluminum pots.*
- *Cook at low heats.*
- *Roast, steam, grill, broil or sauté—don't fry your foods!*

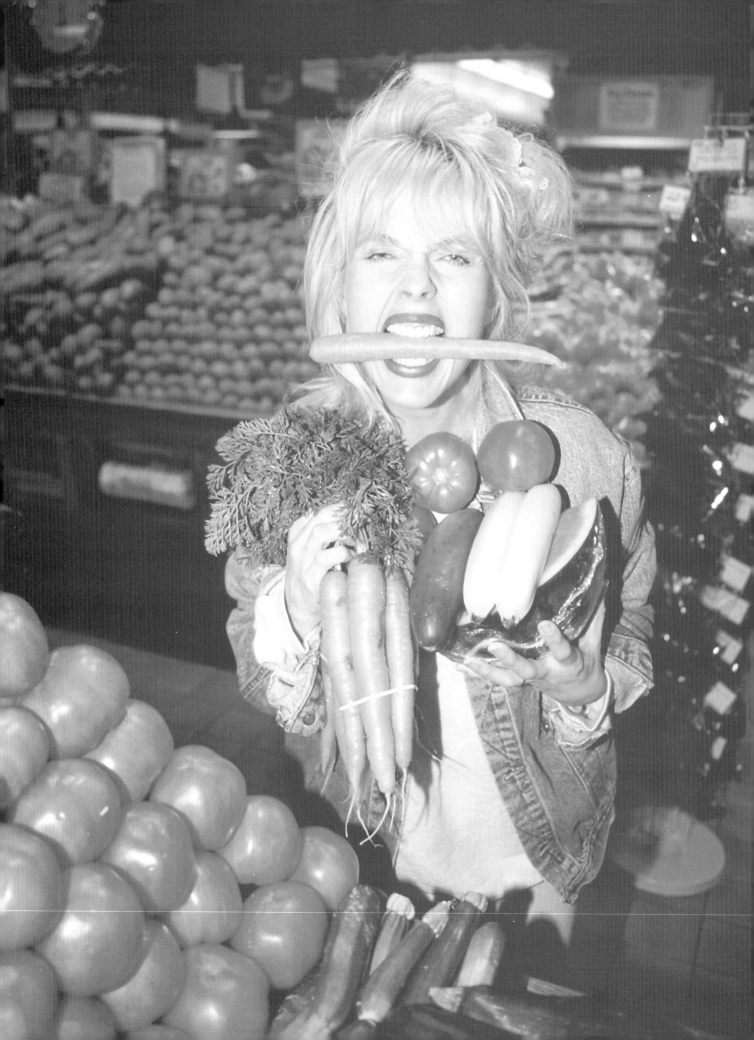

CHAPTER THREE

The Body Under Siege

Scientists continue to uncover the undeniable link between diet and health. Some people ignore the relationship between poor diet and disease, but for others it has provided a basis for a common sense approach to a healthier lifestyle. Over a period spanning forty years, a person is likely to consume approximately 42,000 meals. Isn't it reasonable to suggest that all this food may have a cumulative effect on your overall health?

The food you eat has a profound impact on the very substance of life: your blood, the river of life to your cells. Mucus-producing foods, particularly meat and dairy products, leave behind a residue not unlike the discharge you experience when blowing your nose. This mucus collects throughout your body in tissues, organs, glands and arteries, and over the years, it slowly clogs up the body in the same way dirt and rust plug up a car radiator. When your body is finally overloaded with mucus, you become more vulnerable to an unpleasant array of health problems, such as colds and sore throat, boils, ear infections, pneumonia, fatigue, PMS symptoms and pimples. I think it is important to examine those elements of the typical diet that are particularly suspect in matters of health.

Meat and Other Proteins

While it may be unpleasant to discuss, the truth is that flesh is in a state of

*A slightly over-alkaline diet
is considered beneficial in supporting the
immune system's fight against disease.*

decomposition from the moment an animal dies. The high level of uric acid in the meat we eat creates mucus in our bodies. And even the leanest meat is relatively high in fat. There is not a single species, including human beings, that eats fat exclusive of other substances. Eating 1/4 pound of butter by the spoonful does not sound like a pleasant undertaking. But if you eat a 1/2-pound T-bone steak, only 25% of those calories are providing you with protein. The remaining 75% weighs in as fat.

I feel so much healthier and happier since I stopped eating meat, and believe it is important to my health in general. This intuitive feeling is confirmed by medical research which concludes that meat is directly linked to arterial heart disease and cancer—primary killers in the United States. Hormonal and antibiotic substances which are present in a cow's bloodstream can affect a meat consumer's mental and emotional state as well as his health. If you eat flesh from animals that have been raised on hormones and fed antibiotics and unnatural foods, you are taking a risk with your health. I have abstained from consuming this type of food for many years, because I feel it provides very low quality nutrition and has undesirable effects on my entire digestive system.

As meat begins to decompose, bacteria, uric acid and even worms or parasites are frequently present. Inside your colon, small "pockets" in the colon wall often contain large amounts of the residue from meat products, including these living worms or parasites. A clean, vegetarian diet will tend to cleanse the colon walls and kill these freeloaders, but they are quite content to subsist on unhealthy foods and meat products if allowed to do so. If you undergo colon hydrotherapy, it is not unusual to pass worms or parasites out in your stool. As unpleasant as it is to consider these potential health risks, the consequences of ignoring them are worse than any lack of delicacy in discussion.

The Acid-Alkaline Connection

As the body digests or "burns" its food intake, it leaves behind an ash that is acid, alkaline or neutral. If too many acid residues are left behind in the body tissue, the result is acidosis which is a major cause of many diseases, particularly arthritic conditions. A slightly over-alkaline diet is considered beneficial in supporting the immune system's fight against disease.

- *alkali-forming foods:* dried fruits such as figs, apricots and raisins; pineapple, peaches, bananas; buckwheat and millet; cabbage, watercress, spinach, all vegetable and fruit juices
- *neutral foods:* milk products, vegetable oils

With research and effort,
you can make a lifelong habit
of consuming protein from plant sources.

• *acid-forming foods:* most fish, most meat, most grains, most nuts except almonds and Brazil nuts, lentils

The Benefits of a Vegetarian Diet

Many former meat eaters report increased endurance since becoming vegetarians. An alkaline vegetarian diet has a greater neutralizing effect on the system, thereby extending endurance. Also, meat eaters often experience offensive underarm odors and bad breath, and they may need strong deodorants and mouthwashes to camouflage this unpleasant side effect of meat consumption.

Finally, there is the fundamental matter of raising animals for slaughter. There is no real need to eat secondhand protein which comes from a dead animal. I reached a point where I was uncomfortable lending support, fiscal or otherwise, to the meat industry. With research and effort, you can make a lifelong habit of consuming protein from plant sources. If you think about it, why eat something dead to support your life?

I know it can seem like a daunting task to take meat out of your diet, but in time you lose your taste for it. Eggs are also very hard on the body, tending to cause constipation even more readily than meat. The protein source in eggs is in the egg white. Egg yolks are high in fat.

How about Eggless Egg Salad?

6 oz. firm tofu	1/2 tsp. vegetable oil
1/4 tsp. minced onion	1 tsp. tahini
1/8 cup finely diced celery	1 tbsp. chopped dill or sweet pickle
1/4 tsp. turmeric (for lovely color)	

In a medium bowl, crumble tofu into small pieces. Combine with other ingredients. Season to taste

Delicious on toast or with crackers!

A Word About Grains

Grain products, especially the bleached, processed flours from which we make most of our breads, cereals, pastas, cakes and cookies, cause the body to produce large quantities of mucus and acidic by-products. Think back to childhood play: white flour and water make a very strong paste. Consider the demand that such a paste makes upon the digestive system. Bran, graham, rye or whole wheat are better for you because they lack that paste-like property.

The body manufactures its own cholesterol
which is vital to the execution
of many bodily functions.

The Good... The Bad... The Cholesterol

Cholesterol is produced in the liver and is a raw material in the creation of such things as hormones and cell membranes. Cholesterol is transported in the bloodstream in low-density lipoproteins (LDL), otherwise known as "bad cholesterol" because of its significance in the increased risk of heart attack. Cholesterol that is being released from dead cells is transported in high-density lipoproteins (HDL) and has come to be known as "good cholesterol" for its role in lowering the risk of heart attack. Studies have shown that when the presence of vitamin C in the blood is increased, HDL ("good" cholesterol) levels rise and LDL ("bad" cholesterol) levels decline.

Fat & Cholesterol

There is no doubt that a diet high in saturated fats is a leading factor in the development of coronary heart disease. The major culprits are fatty substances known as cholesterol and triglycerides. The body manufactures its own cholesterol which is vital to the execution of many bodily functions.

Many of the foods we eat also contain cholesterol which is absorbed into the bloodstream during digestion. When there is too much cholesterol present in the blood, that excess is slowly deposited onto the inner walls of the arteries. Gradually, as the inside diameter of the arteries becomes smaller and smaller, the condition known as hardening of the arteries occurs. When a narrowed coronary artery is blocked completely, the heart muscle itself is deprived of the oxygen-rich blood it needs to perform its pumping function. Finally, a heart attack occurs.

Statistics compiled to track people suffering from heart disease indicate that in places where people are more affluent and can afford to eat a high proportion of "fancy foods" like dairy products, eggs, beef and pork—all of which are high in saturated fats—higher rates of heart disease and high cholesterol levels are recorded. It is a dietary pattern that begins in childhood and adolescence, so it is important to avoid eating these foods right from the start. The risk of heart attack is highest in middle-aged and older men, but it is also very high among post-menopausal women.

It is important to mention that we all require a modest amount of fat in our diet. It is when we consume too many fats and oils of the "wrong" kind that we experience health problems. The use of polyunsaturated fats tend to lower the cholesterol level in the blood. I encourage you to eat other

If you include animal products in your diet, choose fish, fat-free milk and dairy products and low-fat cheeses.

foods containing healthy fats, like raw seeds and nuts, unrefined (raw) or cold-pressed vegetable oils and ripe avocados.

If you include animal products in your diet, choose fish, fat-free milk and dairy products and low-fat cheeses. Use only lean cuts of beef, veal, chicken and turkey. Cut away all visible fat, including the skin, before you cook the meat. These simple steps will lower your intake of saturated fats.

USDA Survey of Top Ten Fat Sources Consumed by Americans

margarine	ground beef
whole milk	low-fat milk
shortening	eggs
mayonnaise and salad dressing	butter
American cheese	vanilla ice cream

Cow's Milk and Milk Products

Sometime in your life, you have probably been told that milk is good for you, and that you will grow strong, healthy teeth and bones if you drink lots of it. In recent years, cow's milk has received much intense scrutiny in both the media and medical literature. Research has shown it to be too rich in protein to utilize effectively. It is also very acidic and produces a great deal of mucus.

I drank nearly one-half gallon of milk daily until I was eleven years old. Into my early twenties I continued to drink at least a quart of milk a day. Nevertheless, my teeth have been a weak point in my overall health. My brothers and sisters, on the other hand, disliked milk and never drank much of it, but they have always had strong teeth and few cavities. By the time I was 13, I had fifteen cavities, and I have had many additional cavities filled since then and several of my teeth required crowns.

Cow's milk is intended to make a 25-pound calf grow into a 700-pound animal in four to five months. To achieve this end, cow's milk is loaded with natural growth hormones that are good for a calf's body but inappropriate to the human body. Many people suffer from indigestion and even allergic reactions to cow's milk. Today, there is the additional

If you continue to eat dairy products,
do so in moderation and along with raw green
vegetables to aid digestion and assimilation.

complication of artificial additives in milk. Our dairy animals receive numerous injections of antibiotics because, due to substandard living conditions, they are frequently sick. In order to make the cows produce a bountiful supply of milk year-round, the dairy farmer may inject them with synthetic hormones as well. When you drink milk, you also take these dangerous hormones and unnecessary antibiotics into your body.

If you are concerned about obtaining sufficient calcium, there are many alternate sources. Dark green vegetables like kale, broccoli and collard greens, as well as nuts, seeds and dried fruit, are wonderful sources of calcium. If you are worried about protein intake, "milks" from sesame seeds, almonds and numerous other seeds and nuts are much better for your body and supply plentiful protein. Blended with dates and bananas, they make a delicious "milk" shake. Soy and rice milk are available in any good health food store. They come in many flavors and varieties and can be substituted for cow's milk in your diet. From all the information I have read on milk since becoming a vegetarian, it is clear to me that it is better to avoid pasteurized milk and all of its products. I avoid all dairy products except an occasional pat of raw butter. Remember that raw, unpasteurized dairy products are easier to digest because they still contain live enzymes. If you continue to eat dairy products, do so in moderation and along with raw green vegetables to aid digestion and assimilation.

Salt

I know many people who cannot savor their food unless they put lots of salt on it, but salt actually masks subtle food flavors. If you stop using salt, your taste buds will once again become more sensitive, and food will begin to have distinct flavors. Like cigarettes, salt inhibits your taste buds as you get older, and that takes the fun out of eating. Salt and various condiments, many of which contain high quantities of salt, can irritate, damage and even poison the cells of the tissues, organs and glands as they travel through the body via the bloodstream. Salt causes cells of the tissues and organs to harden and is one of the causes of high blood pressure, heart disease and rheumatism. Excess salt contributes to dry and wrinkled skin. Salt consumption leads to increased thirst and water consumption, resulting in bloat and a water-logged body. Water retention retards the elimination of toxic salts from the body.

In most restaurants, chefs put salt on food to make it more appetizing. This is especially true of meat dishes, so beware! Specify that your food have no salt added or choose foods with low salt contents when eating out.

At home, pass up canned and frozen vegetable items which have salt added.

The Front Line in the Battle Against Salt

Freshly picked or dried and crumbled, herbs have been used for centuries by experienced chefs. Fresh herbs can be successfully refrigerated if you wrap them in a damp wash cloth or dish towel and then store the herbs in a plastic bag. If you choose to use dried herbs, one teaspoon is roughly the equivalent of one tablespoon of the fresh variety.

- *Basil:* Highly aromatic and fundamental to Italian cooking. Excellent in sauces or with mildly flavored vegetables such as zucchini. One or two fresh leaves roughly cut are delicious in a green salad.
- *Bay Leaf:* One dried leaf is enough for a whole pot of veggie stew. A savory element in a sweet and sour sauce. Be careful not to overdo it.
- *Dill:* Here is the taste you love in dill pickles. This tart but delicate herb is the perfect subtle compliment to yogurt for a refreshing dip or salad dressing.
- *Rosemary:* Roasted with potatoes and carrots, this savory herb will fill the house with its delicious, earthy aroma. Best used fresh by the sprig in soups or stews. It will hold together on its wood-like stalk and is best removed before serving.
- *Sage:* The flavor of beans, potatoes and all root vegetables is enhanced by this subtle flavor. An excellent companion to the more pungent taste of rosemary.
- *Sweet Marjoram:* A discreet cousin to its better known cousin, oregano. Use it to add subtlety to old favorites like minestrone soup. Sprinkle over slices of garden fresh tomatoes.
- *Tarragon:* A vivid, fragrant herb, vital to much classic French cooking. Use it to flavor vinegar. An unexpected licorice flavor best used lightly with vegetables or grains.

At home, pass up canned and frozen vegetable items which have salt added. You need not worry that you'll deny yourself necessary salt. It is present in just about every cake, bread, cookie, sauce and dairy product. Even candy is salted! Try making the effort to look for unsalted, natural products from health food stores or the natural food section of your supermarket. Always read labels! Ingredients are listed on the side panels of most products. Learn

Try making the effort to look for unsalted,
natural products from health food stores
or the natural food section of your supermarket.
Always read labels!

what an acceptable daily total of fat and salt is for your body. People often realize how addicted they are to salt and condiments when they attempt to eliminate these items from their diet. Buy some salt-free ketchup, and if the taste doesn't appeal to you, experiment by adding your own herbs and spices. Food may taste flat to you without salt, but moderation is always an option. If you're not prepared to go completely salt-free, then try using less salt. Have patience while your taste buds repair themselves, and food will display far more variety and subtlety than you thought possible.

A Sugar Is a Sugar Is a Sugar!

By FDA standards, sugarless and sugar-free products do not contain sucrose. But watch out! Dextrose, sorbitol, xylitol, mannitol, glucose, galactose and maltose all contain sugar.

Eliminating Refined Sugar

Sugar, a refined carbohydrate, represents the ultimate in empty, non-nutritious calories. It clogs the system, overwhelming the digestive organs and affecting the brain. If you are already suffering from digestive problems, it is especially important to refrain from sugar. Sugary foods frequently trigger a sour stomach because they ferment in the digestive system. When a body is overwhelmed by overconsumption of sugar, it can develop hypoglycemia, a condition characterized by the body's inability to properly metabolize sugar. Symptoms such as dizziness, fatigue, headache, restlessness and confusion can be subtle or acute. Psychological and emotional problems like anxiety and depression have also been linked to sugar consumption.

It was actually easier than I thought it would be to give up sugary foods. My new diet contained so many fresh and dried fruits that whenever I had a craving for something sweet, I bought dried figs, dates, pineapple or papaya slices. These became my favorite "candy." All the fresh fruit drinks on my program also went a long way in satisfying my cravings for sweets.

One of the most important tips I can pass along to you is to find out which of the dried fruits is most satisfying to your sweet tooth, and make sure you have some on hand! If you stalk around your kitchen desperate for something sweet, you are likely to find yourself munching on a chocolate bar from the corner store before you even realize you're there. But the immediate gratification of a handful of sweet dates is surprisingly satisfying. When you

Tasteless "health food"
is a thing of the past.

get the urge for a candy bar, biting into a crunchy apple may not make it, but dried, succulent papaya or pineapple fit the bill with sweet, chewy success. There is a new world of choices in healthy sweets, from "shakes" to cakes. Tasteless "health food" is a thing of the past. There are absolutely delicious juice-sweetened cookies that even your children will enjoy. Experiment until you find some healthy sweets for that instant gratification you've come to identify with sugar. Your vigilance will be well rewarded.

Systems Overloaded with Mucus

The amount of white mucus present on your tongue is an indication of your prevailing "mucus condition." Look at your tongue in the mirror before you brush your teeth. The more white mucus coating your tongue, the more clogged with mucus you can expect your whole body to be. Just as cholesterol clogs arteries and veins, mucus clogs organs and other areas with similar results. Together with other toxins and excess fats from the average American diet, mucus breaks down our systems. If we fail to halt that process by cleansing our bodies of all the accumulated waste matter, we will most probably end up with some kind of illness. The minute we stop putting all the wrong foods into our bodies, we start to eliminate the impurities that have collected inside us since we were babies. Gradually we start feeling better and looking better. After all, "You are what you eat!"

Toxic Relief

As cleansers and builders, fruits and vegetables produce no mucus and contain elements for producing vital energy and life-supporting components which are superior to those in any other foods. These elements and ingredients are known as organized carbon and "grape sugar." Fruits and vegetables have all the tissue salts needed by the body. You may decide you want more culinary variety in your life, but simply put, fruits and vegetables offer all the good news with none of the bad.

A Look into the Future on a Mucus-Free Diet

Let's say you've taken steps to improve your diet and been happy with the results. Now you're really motivated and you want to see what this mucus-free diet is all about. You've looked back over your food journal and you know a lot about your strengths and vulnerabilities with regard to various foods. You decide to take the plunge and try a mucus-free diet for two months. You go through your kitchen tossing out some obvious enemies and stocking up on the foods that will be your allies in this experiment.

When your body is no longer overtaxed
by the need to rid itself of toxins and mucus,
it can direct its available energy to healing.

Your new diet will rely upon fruits, vegetables, seeds and nuts—all of them mucus- and toxin-free. You know that your body will go through a deep cleansing while continuing to be fed with all the vitamins, minerals and beneficial nutrients it needs. As the debris from mucus-rich foods is eliminated from your system, the beneficial effects of a healthy diet will be revealed.

You will begin to feel stronger and more energized. Your eyes will be brighter and you might even experience improved eyesight. Your sinus passages and lungs will be clear. If adult acne was a problem, it will improve and perhaps disappear. After several weeks on this diet, you'll notice a marked decrease of earwax. Your breath will definitely be sweeter. You will experience less perspiration and odor under your arms, and you may be able to discontinue the use of deodorants. In fact, you will note much less body odor in general. Any tendency toward "bloatedness" will be gone. Your skin will look younger and take on a rosy glow and surface wrinkles will diminish.

Overall, your vitality, endurance and energy level will be dramatically increased. After a while, your hair and nails will grow more quickly and look healthier. Your thinking will be more focused and you'll need less sleep. You'll likely find it easier to stay optimistic and positive about yourself and the world around you. PMS symptoms will be minimized. When your body is no longer overtaxed by the need to rid itself of toxins and mucus, it can direct its available energy to healing. Colds will not linger, injuries will heal more rapidly. This is an extra benefit of letting the body detoxify itself naturally. The constant strengthening of the body and building up of its immune system is an important factor in fighting disease.

Finally, this new standard of healthy eating will be the catalyst that drives your body to seek its ideal weight. Now you are truly motivated and your continued commitment to eating well and feeling great has become your greatest ally in the battle to maintain that weight.

Mucus-Free Diet and Good Health

After years on a mucus-free diet, I feel that most of the foods we usually eat are like poisons wrapped in very attractive packages. While we pride ourselves on our external appearances, a high degree of internal physical uncleanness has unfortunately become the norm. Autopsies routinely reveal the extent of internal plaque and waste retained by the intestines and colon. Most people live in this state of uncleanness without even realizing it, even though the foul odor of their bowels and bad breath are indications of this prevailing impurity.

I know that the mucus-free diet is not for everyone. But I have tried all

I can promise you that whatever degree of commitment you make to healthier eating, your body will pay you back in kind.

kinds of different diets over the years and there is no doubt in my mind that the mucus-free diet is the superior one for me. The way I feel and the way I look when I stay on it for extended periods shows me this is the right way. It absolutely slows down the body's aging process. It is rare for people to guess my real age and they usually think I am ten years younger. While I don't fear growing older, I am happy to have the vitality that makes people mistake me for a younger woman. Please understand that no one knows better than I the kind of commitment needed to follow such a pure food program. Even after years of study and experimentation, I struggle to live up to my own standard of dietary health. I would never suggest that this is easy. But I can promise you that whatever degree of commitment you make to healthier eating, your body will pay you back in kind.

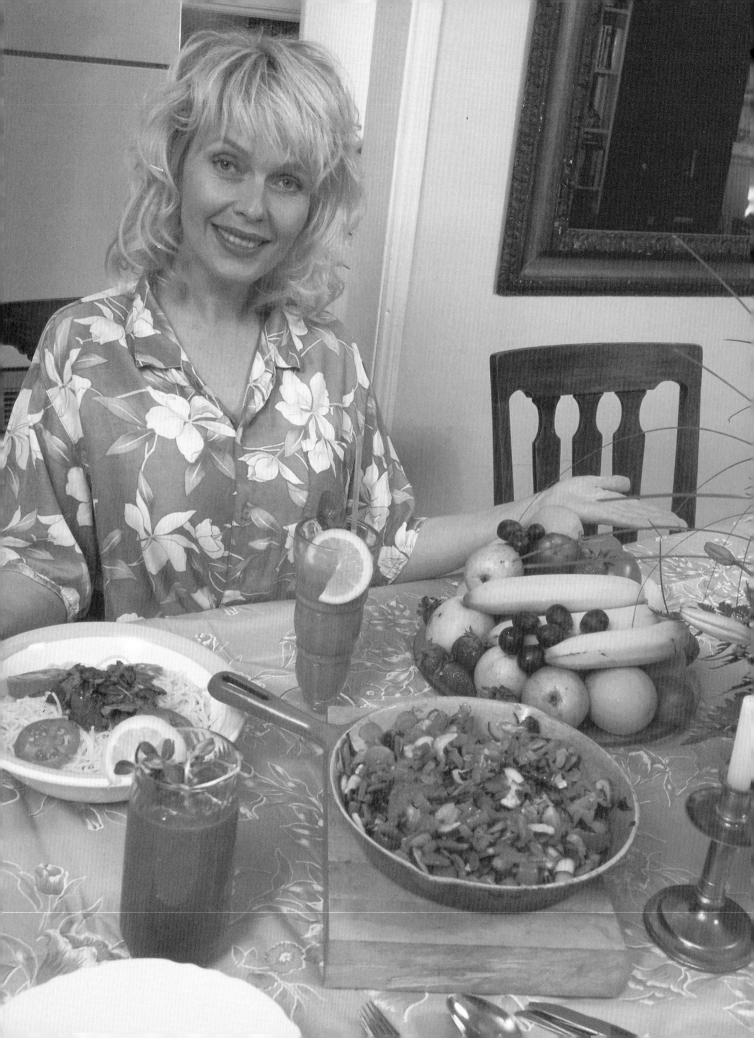

CHAPTER FOUR

Recipes

I am going to give you some of my favorite recipes. They contain both raw and cooked ingredients. They are all healthy and good for you, but I prefer the raw food most of the time.

Juices, Smoothies, Shakes & Sorbets

Pineapple Juice: Cut up a pineapple and put it through a juicer. That's all you do, and it makes delicious juice. If you experience periodic water retention or want to lose a few pounds, this is a wonderful way to go!

Pineapple/Strawberry Juice: Juice strawberries and pineapple together.

Orange/Strawberry Juice: Put orange sections and strawberries through the juicer.

Orange/Banana Smoothie: Squeeze oranges and put the juice in a blender. Add bananas, preferably frozen ones. This drink is great tasting and fills you up. It helps you shed pounds because it contains no fat, is highly nutritious, and gives you that "full" feeling.

Apple/Strawberry Juice: Cut your apples up and put them through your juicer. Pour the apple juice into your blender and add some strawberries.

Apple/Raspberry Juice: Same as Apple/Strawberry Juice, but substitute raspberries.

Apple/Celery/Almond Drink: Cut up apples and celery in equal amounts

Melon and melon juice should be eaten alone or left alone. Remember that advice.

before juicing them. Transfer the juice to a blender and add 15 to 20 blanched almonds and some ice. Blend until smooth. This is a very refreshing, nourishing drink and it's very tasty.

Apple/Carrot Juice: Juice equal amounts of apples and carrots. They taste great together, and provide lots of vitamins and minerals.

Lemonade: Squeeze fresh lemons manually and add maple syrup to the juice to taste. Dilute with distilled water and chill. This wonderful drink is refreshing and very cleansing.

From time to time, you might also wish to drink a cup of this warm with a pinch of cayenne pepper, for extra cleansing purposes. Many people live on this drink for days to cleanse their bodies and restore themselves to good health.

Wheat Grass Juice: Many people feel this is the most health-promoting food in the world. They swear that it can cure all kinds of diseases and other physical problems. It contains all the vitamins, minerals and amino acids necessary to feed and cleanse the body. Many health food stores sell fresh wheat grass juice that they make from flats of fresh, growing wheat grass.

To make wheat grass juice at home, you need a special juicer designed especially to process wheat grass. I have used a manual one, but it takes a lot of effort to make it work. Although an electric one costs approximately $200, I recommend this type because it is much easier to use.

A daily intake of one to six ounces of wheat grass juice is recommended. I usually drink two ounces. You can drink it "straight" or add it to carrot or other mixed vegetable juices.

Melon Juice: Cut up any type of ripe melon flesh and put it through your juicer. Melon is almost 100% water and very good for you. I find watermelon juice the most tasty, and all melon juices are superb cleansers. Experiment with juicing seeds, rinds and all. Melon and melon juice should be eaten alone or left alone. Remember that advice.

Grape Juice: Put any kind of fresh grapes through a juicer. The result is one of the most nourishing, cleansing drinks in the world!

Celery/Zucchini/Carrot Juice: Put one half carrot, one quarter zucchini and one quarter celery (2:1 by proportion) through the juicer. This is a very refreshing and healthy drink.

Carrot juice is a great source of vitamin A and it can help boost immunity.

Beet/Carrot Juice: Prepare six ounces carrot juice and two ounces beet juice (3:1 by proportion) and combine for a very "earthy" tasting drink. Beet juice is very concentrated when extracted and goes a long way in combination with other juices because of its strong flavor. I love this drink! It is a wonderful blood builder too.

Carrot/Beet/Celery/Parsley Drink: This is a very nourishing combination! Juice mainly carrots with a small amount of beet, celery and parsley. Parsley has an overpowering taste but it is very good for you. It contains lots of chlorophyll, iron and calcium. Celery juice is said to be good for the nerves and for many bodily functions. Carrot juice, by the way, is a great source of vitamin A and it can help boost immunity. I use it as the base of every vegetable drink I make.

Carrot/Celery/Spinach Drink: Juice mainly carrots, then add celery and spinach to taste. This is a very cleansing, blood-building drink.

Carrot/Cucumber/Beet Juice: Juice mainly carrots with one cucumber and a small amount of beets.

Celery/Apple Juice: Juice in half and half proportions. This tasty drink is good for balancing the body.

Celery/Carrot/Apple Juice: Juice almost equal parts, with extra carrots. A holistic doctor prescribed this drink for me once when I was not feeling well. I drank it once a day and drank Apple/Carrot Juice the rest of the time for three days. It worked wonders to cleanse my system and restore my health.

Pineapple/Mango Juice: Juice a pineapple with one mango. This is one of my favorite drinks.

Pineapple/Papaya Juice: Juice a pineapple with one papaya. I drank this juice every day for over a year, and it is still a favorite of mine. Papayas are helpful to the digestive system. I drank it often when I was pregnant because this mixture contains a lot of calcium.

Apple/Peach/Banana Smoothie: Juice apples and transfer the liquid to a blender. Add peach and banana to taste. This is another tasty and filling drink.

Almond milk with a whole grain cereal,
neither of which has added sugar or salt,
is a superior substitute for cow's milk
and processed, sugary cereals.

Apple/Raspberry/Banana Smoothie: Same as Apple/Raspberry Juice, but add frozen bananas. The result is thick and sweet. My daughter loves this one!

Apple/Peach/Banana Smoothie: Juice apples and transfer the liquid to a blender. Add peach and banana to taste. This is another tasty and filling drink. Frozen, whole raw bananas give your drinks a thick, creamy texture. If you freeze them on a stick, they make delicious healthy treats. Peel very ripe bananas when there is no green on the skin and brown spots have begun to appear. Freeze them ten to twelve at a time in a plastic bag. I make banana smoothies every day. Bananas also add sweetness to drinks when they are blended with almost any fruit. You can add raw sesame seeds or fresh shredded coconut to any of these fruit drinks. These additions give your smoothie an even smoother consistency. Of course, they add healthy oils and extra protein and minerals as well. Sesame seeds are especially high in calcium.

Almond Milk Shake: My daughter and I drink a delightful "milk shake" made in a blender. Use one cup of almonds, four cups of water, add dates and vanilla extract to taste. Soak the almonds overnight and drain that water off. Put the almonds into the blender and add more water. Blend well and strain the mixture through a fine mesh strainer. Return the liquid to the blender, add vanilla and dates and blend a final time. This is a great "milk." It is tasty and healthy and will not make you fat. I promise! I drink it straight or pour it over cereal. Almond milk with a whole grain cereal, neither of which has added sugar or salt, is a superior substitute for cow's milk and processed, sugary cereals. Personally, I think the healthy choice tastes better. It puts no undesirable fats, cholesterol, mucus or acid-forming elements into your system. My daughter loves this dish.

Sesame, Sunflower Seed and/or Cashew Milks: Each of these has a distinct flavor so try them all to find out what you like best. Make sure the nuts and seeds you use are raw and unsalted. Instead of dates, you can use raisins, dried figs, dried apricots or peaches to sweeten the "milk." In my experience, dates give the best flavor. If the dried fruit has been soaked overnight, it purées more easily.

Fruit Sorbets—Home Preparation

Everybody seems to like ice cream, but it contains large amounts of cow's milk, sugar and unhealthy additives and fillers. Fruit freezes and sorbets made at

Bean and pea sprouts make particularly good, quick snacks.

home do not have these unwanted ingredients. You can make a variety of flavors from many kinds of seasonally available fruits, especially bananas. Freeze the fruits after you have sliced them. You need a Champion juicer or blender to assist you in this process.

Pear/Banana Sorbet: Put pear slices in the blender and add banana to taste. To make the mixture combine more easily, add a little apple juice. For added sweetness, toss in a few fresh dates.

Use the same procedure to make these flavors:
• *Grape/Banana*
• *Strawberry/Banana*
• *Banana/Strawberry/Pineapple*
• *Banana/Peach/Nectarine/Grape*
• *Banana/Papaya/Mango/Kiwi*

Experiment! Use your imagination! Freeze all your favorite fruits in any combination. They will all come out well and you can develop some exotic treats for your guests. You will love the taste of your sorbets and they are very cleansing. You know they are very nourishing when you make them yourself. They contain no mucus-or acid-forming dairy products or fat! Eat these homemade sorbets all day long, and you will not gain a gram. Splurge!

Veggies, Soups, Sandwiches, Stews

Salad in a Blender or "Energy Soup": This wonderful mixture is tasty and enormously good for you. It is one of the most nutritious soups in the world! Cut up and put in the blender one medium tomato, one half cucumber, a handful of alfalfa sprouts, several romaine lettuce and spinach leaves and one stalk of celery, and then squeeze half a lemon over it. Blend until it is puréed together and looks like "soup." Add one half avocado, kelp or dulse for extra flavor, if desired.

There are many varieties of green sprouts which can be substituted for alfalfa sprouts. The most common are buckwheat, clover, radish, sunflower and onion sprouts. Bean and pea sprouts are also good, as are lentils. Sprouts of this kind contain fantastic food value and contain essential nutrients like chlorophyll, protein, vitamins and minerals. Even when you are not making "energy soup," add them to your sandwiches and salads and as a garnish on your dinner plate. Bean and pea sprouts make particularly good, quick snacks. They supply your body with rich fuel for the day.

If you eat cayenne that has been brought to a boil, it will act as an internal irritant, so do not add it to soup that you expect to reheat.

Vegetable Soup or Stew: My absolute favorite soup can be made with slightly less water to take on a "stew" consistency or it can be puréed. Sauté celery, onion and garlic over low heat in a small amount of unrefined vegetable oil. Use just the amount of oil needed to prevent the vegetables from sticking to your pan. I prefer olive, safflower or peanut oil. Add chopped carrots, different squashes, potatoes, cauliflower, fresh green peas, broccoli, rutabaga— plus any other vegetables you like! Add one pint water, more or less, depending on how concentrated you want the cooked mixture to become. Cook 45 minutes to one hour. When all the vegetables have cooked completely, add kelp or dulse and/or fresh lemon juice to taste. If you like, add cayenne pepper to individual portions just before serving. If you eat cayenne that has been brought to a boil, it will act as an internal irritant, so do not add it to soup that you expect to reheat.

Guacamole Sandwich: Use big leaves of lettuce, the bigger the better, in place of two slices of bread. Mash an avocado adding very finely chopped tomato, cucumber, celery, onion, cilantro and a few drops of freshly squeezed lemon juice. For additional flavor to taste, add a tiny bit of cayenne pepper, Jensen's Dry Vegetable Seasoning, or Bragg's Liquid amino (no-salt soy sauce). Spread your creation between the two lettuce leaves and eat it like a sandwich. This is my favorite sandwich. It tastes fantastic, has a lot of nutrients and will never make you fat.

Chinese Vegetables: In a wok or large frying pan, heat a small amount (approx. 1 tbsp.) of vegetable oil, preferably sesame or peanut. Stir in chopped celery, onion, garlic and ginger root and cook for a minute. Add 1/2 - 1 cup of water, then chopped cauliflower, broccoli, Chinese pea pods, different squashes and water chestnuts. Cook approx. 5 minutes. Add bean sprouts and cut firm tofu chunks if you like more protein with this dish. Cook approx. 2 minutes more. After cooking, stir in a touch of fresh lemon juice, cayenne pepper or Bragg's Liquid Amino if you prefer a saltier flavor. Serve with brown rice.

French Bakes: I have told you about my favorite potato dish before, but I want to mention it especially here. Cut raw potatoes into thin strips like regular potato chips or french fries. Spread the strips out on a non-stick cookie sheet. Bake in an oven preheated to 425° until they are light brown. Turn them over and brown the other side. These potatoes taste

Dried fruits of all kinds make quick,
easy, nutritious snacks.

great plain or with no salt, sugar-free ketchup. Their great taste is not overwhelmed by fats or oils, so they have relatively few calories and you can eat lots of them.

Fruits

Dried Fruits: Dried fruits of all kinds make quick, easy, nutritious snacks. I eat lots of them. My daughter eats them instead of sugary candies. I soak them overnight, which restores their plumpness. Make sure to buy dry fruits in their unsulfured form. Sulfur is an irritant to your bloodstream and can be dangerous to people who suffer from allergies.

Fresh Apple Sauce: Cook apples just until you can mash them. Add a touch of lemon juice and a few raisins. My daughter loves this one, and so do I.

Frozen Bananas: Peel ripe bananas when brown spots begin to appear. Insert a stick in each, and then freeze the bananas. This makes a great healthy treat for a hot day.

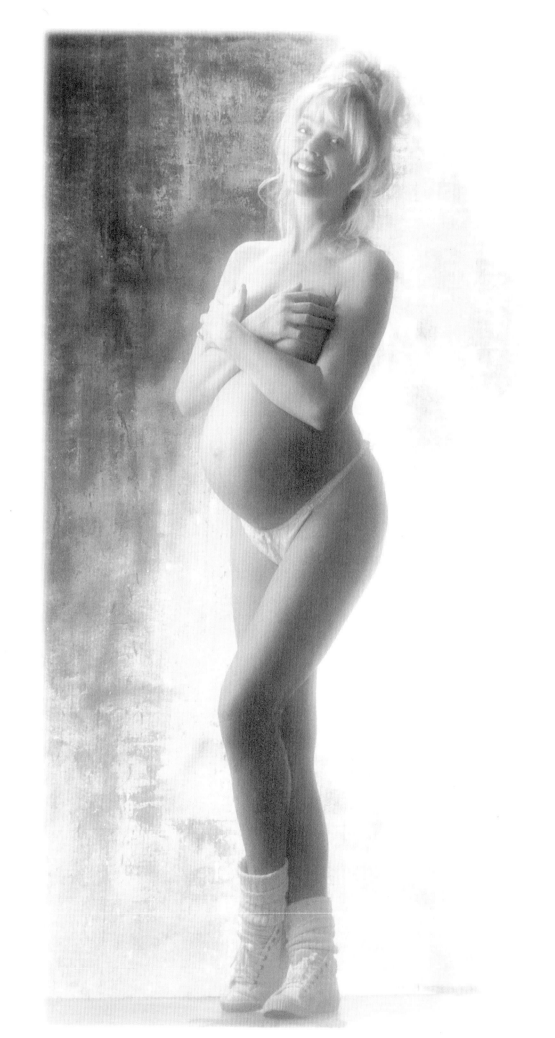

CHAPTER FIVE

My Pregnancy Experience

Since becoming pregnant and having my child, I've met many women in their late thirties and well into their forties who are having babies. Some are adding second or third children to the family and others, like me, waited to have their first. Pregnancy was a thrilling challenge for me, and I rose to meet it with enthusiasm.

My pregnancy came as a surprise and I was at once extremely happy and full of worries and questions. I had not been making preparations, so there was much I needed to learn. Fortunately, I was very healthy and in fine physical condition. I had been exercising and eating well for years. Even though I was chronologically in my late thirties, I felt more like a person ten years younger in body and mind. Due to my positive frame of mind, my healthy diet and regular exercise, I had reached a point in my life travels where I knew that my chronological age was not an indication of my physical and mental age. As I've said many times, I strongly believe if you take good care of yourself and live right, you will stay young and healthy in mind and body all your life. I am aware of how important your mental attitude is to your overall health, and so I have aged much more slowly than most others my age. My pregnancy was a perfect opportunity to live out my belief, and I am happy to say that now, four years after a happy, healthy pregnancy, I'm in even better overall condition than I was ten years ago.

Listen to your body!
It will tell you when to slow down
and when to stop.

Exercising My Body and My Mind

As a vegetarian, I have been wonderfully healthy and have not had any cause to take medication or see a physician. When I was pregnant with my daughter, I went to a doctor for regular check-ups. Happily, my pregnancy was quite easy and I had no complications. I underwent natural childbirth, free of all medications. I am happy to say that since my daughter's birth, I have had no further need for a physician or any prescription medications. Both my young daughter and I are in excellent health. She has been a vegetarian since birth, of course.

For the most part, I really was ready for my pregnancy even though it was a surprise. With the consent and support of my doctor, I resolved to continue with some form of exercise into my third trimester. For the first three months of the pregnancy, I exercised in much the same way I always had. My routine consisted of using an exercycle for an average of 45 minutes daily. In addition, I walked up and down steps for 20 minutes three times a week, went to the gym three times a week and did a 40-minute routine with free weights and Nautilus equipment. I also stretched every day and did side twists with a stick to keep my waist firm. It is very important to note that this exercise regimen was one I had been following for many years, and I continued with my regimen only with my doctor's consent. Pregnancy is not the time for an unconditioned woman to begin a program of strenuous exercise or diet modification.

As I entered my second trimester, I was feeling great. I continued to exercise but cut my first trimester routine by half, and began to take long walks every day.

During the final trimester, I stopped going to the gym, and again, with the consent of my doctor, did a gentle floor routine and used the exercycle in moderation. I climbed steps for shorter time periods and worked on my upper arms with five-pound weights. I took each day as it came and let my body tell me when to slow down or stop.

The last month, I concentrated mostly on walking. I believe in keeping the blood circulation going strong by doing a light amount of exercise with periodic rest. Most importantly, do not exhaust yourself by exercising too much. I found swimming and walking to be the perfect exercises toward the end of my pregnancy. Listen to your body! It will tell you when to slow down and when to stop.

Frequently throughout the day I would take a few moments to rest, play soft music, think joyful thoughts and make a space for peace and harmony within myself. I join many pregnant women in the belief that our unborn children can sense all that good energy coming their way. Whether

*The more oxygen you can bring to your body,
the better your body can assimilate nutrients
and the clearer your thinking will be.*

or not an unborn child is capable of sensing its mother's state of mind, I felt it was important to put my mind to good use. I read biographies about inventors, business moguls and philosophers; or spiritual passages from the Bible and other metaphysical works. It takes very little time to follow a positive and constructive program like this. I know only that it made me happy and peaceful and I believe my baby appreciated that.

Daily Hygiene

I elevated my feet whenever necessary to prevent water retention in my legs. Deep breathing is something I also did many times daily. The more oxygen you can bring to your body, the better your body can assimilate nutrients and the clearer your thinking will be.

Dry brushing the skin is also very good for you. Get a brush with natural bristles and a long handle so you can reach every part of your back. A couple of minutes a day, preferably before showering, is all it takes. Dry brushing promotes good circulation, improves your glandular system, and helps keep your body feeling clean inside and out. Dead skin cells are whisked away and your skin starts to look nice and rosy. Dry brushing also helps to break up cellulite deposits just under the skin's surface. For more on this technique, see Chapter Eight.

Make sure you get enough sunlight. Natural light gives you energy and strength. The sun's rays stimulate the formation of vitamin D by your body, which aids in the assimilation of calcium, particularly important during pregnancy. Take sunbaths for short periods of time, exposing all of your body if you can. The warmth rejuvenates the skin and helps to eliminate impurities from your system. Too much sunbathing can cause more harm than good, but 30-minute intervals before or after the high heat of the day are fine for most people.

I was concerned about stretch marks and drank plenty of liquids to avoid them. I used a "homemade" moisturizer made from half aloe vera gel and half pure coconut oil. I massaged this mixture into all areas of my skin, paying particular attention to belly, breasts and buttocks. After my child was born, I did not have any stretch marks.

Pregnancy Diet

I was especially careful to stay away from salt and all salty foods in order to prevent water retention. I avoided all white, processed sugar and products with high sugar content because of the detrimental chemical effect sugar has on the body as well as to save unwanted calories. There is very little nutritional value in white flour products and they can cause constipation, so I did

*Your body needs healthy fats and oils
on a regular basis, but you need more of them
when you are pregnant.*

not eat them at all. I did have one gluttonous episode (Remember the sausages in Chapter One?) when I was on holiday in Norway. And I retained the water to prove it. But with the exception of sparing use of raw, unpasteurized butter, I did not use dairy products. Dairy products are too high in concentrated protein, and if not organic, contain residual toxins due to hormones and antibiotics fed to the cows to increase milk production. Of course, I never touched alcohol or cigarettes or any other drugs.

Special Diet Problems in Pregnancy

I ate very well during my pregnancy and never had the problem with constipation that some of my friends experienced. I did make a special effort to prevent constipation, however. I took in two to four quarts of pure water, fresh fruit juices, and fresh vegetable juices daily. The water and juice also flushed toxins from my body and kept my skin looking beautiful. Exercise helped me guard against constipation in my pregnancy as it does throughout my everyday life. My diet consisted almost entirely of raw and cooked fruits and vegetables, with raw nuts—all full of fiber and nutrients.

Pregnant women have an increased need for iron. I soaked dried fruits such as figs, prunes and raisins overnight and blended them into a sweet purée. They satisfied my sweet tooth and had a laxative effect. Many fresh fruits contain iron, especially red berries and bananas. Among the fresh vegetables, beets, leafy greens, wheat grass and sprouts are iron-rich, as are sea vegetables like kelp and dulse. Blackstrap molasses contains concentrated iron.

I was sunbathing to enhance my calcium absorption, but I also consumed calcium by drinking lots of fresh carrot juice mixed with liquefied parsley, spinach and celery. Steamed collard greens, kale and broccoli are also good calcium sources. I ate many papayas. Filberts and pistachio nuts were two of my favorite treats. Kelp and dulse are also high in calcium. I sprinkled them in dehydrated form on my salads and steamed vegetables.

Increased Need for Protein

I made a type of "milk" from sesame seeds and blanched almonds, both of which are high in calcium. Raw carob powder also contains calcium and added a delicious flavor to my nutty "milkshakes." I combined all these ingredients in a blender with some ice. It came out almost like a chocolate smoothie!

Your body needs healthy fats and oils on a regular basis, but you need more of them when you are pregnant. I used raw, extra virgin olive oil on my salad and steamed vegetables, plus slices of ripe avocado. Raw nuts and seeds, nut butters and my nutty "milkshakes" also supplied me with excellent

I can resist everything
except temptation.

Oscar Wilde (1854 - 1900)

Irish-born British dramatist, "Lady Windermere's Fan"

sources of healthy fat.

It is a medical fact that pregnant women have a heightened need for protein during gestation. In my case, the nut/seed milk, vegetables dipped in raw nut butters, and bean and pea sprouts took care of my protein requirements. I also occasionally used raw wheat germ and brewer's yeast in small amounts. Once in a while I ate or drank soy products like soy milk, soy ice cream, soy burgers or soy dogs. Plain tofu was my favorite soy product. I ate it unprepared, straight from the package. It is also good mixed into stews or scrambled with chopped vegetables so that the result is something like an omelet. Now and then I ate beans or peas in a soup or stew, to which I also added barley and other grains to make a complete protein.

Other Food Favorites

One item I ate a lot of was mashed potatoes with a touch of unsalted, raw butter and a bit of ground pepper. I used pepper sparingly because it is known to irritate your bloodstream, but it certainly tasted good on mashed potatoes. My favorite health food store stocks fresh muffins made from whole wheat flour and oat bran. They are sweetened with fruit and contain no eggs or salt. These were high on my list of special treats.

Occasionally I ate a whole wheat pizza with soy cheese. I had a soy burger on very rare occasions, or a soy wiener with unsalted ketchup and mustard on a whole wheat bun. Not the best food combining perhaps, but awfully good to a very pregnant woman!

Cravings!

I ate a limited amount of whole grain and sprouted grain breads and cereals. I actually developed a craving for cereal and soy milk. I used puffed millet, corn or rice and sometimes corn flakes—all without added sugar and salt. I sweetened my dish with a tablespoon or so of maple syrup and truly enjoyed it.

Occasionally, I craved an animal product, so I'd have some fresh salmon or red snapper, and once in a while, I'd have eggs, unpasteurized cheese or butter. These cravings were rare, but they did happen, and I indulged them without tormenting myself with guilt. If I craved something spicy or fried, I'd make baked potato chips. Sometimes I would buy unsalted corn chips and natural salsa (no salt) and sit down to eat a big bag of the chips dipped in salsa while I read a book or watched television.

Bread has always been one of my favorite foods. My mother used to make plump loaves which I loved as a child. Usually I do not eat much of it at one time, but while I was pregnant I constantly craved fresh bread. A loaf

*Be sure to consult your doctor
before taking any vitamin/mineral products.*

of sprouted whole grain bread or a pack of unsalted whole wheat pita pockets satisfied me. I made sure these products contained no salt and little oil. They were good toasted with sliced bananas on top, with unsalted raw butter, fruit jams, or sliced avocado, tomato, cucumber, sprouts and lettuce. I called my various fruit and vegetable combinations my "salad sandwich."

Vitamin/Mineral Supplements

Before I was pregnant, I lived on fresh fruits and salads almost exclusively. During my pregnancy, I could not stay on this program for more than a couple of days at a time. I am convinced by this experience that your body needs more concentrated foodstuffs, starches and proteins when you are pregnant. The cravings I developed were so strong that it felt like my body was talking to me, telling me to eat more foods and different ones than usual.

I started taking a vitamin and mineral supplement after the first few months of pregnancy. One of my teeth had started to loosen, and I certainly did not want to lose it! That was the only health problem I experienced throughout my entire pregnancy. I began to think of that one tooth as a sort of sentry, warning me if I was not getting enough of something. I felt instinctively that I should start taking vitamin and mineral supplements in response. After a few days on my supplement program, the tooth was firm in its socket again. If your gums bleed, as mine did, increase your intake of vitamin C. Floss more often and use the rubber tip on your toothbrush to massage the gums between your teeth. I also massaged my gums with aloe vera gel and rinsed with salt water. Slightly chewed wheat grass pulp placed along your gums several times a day for ten to twenty minutes is very helpful. When I was seven months pregnant, I went to Norway on what turned into a long vacation. I had chosen to use a very powerful vitamin/mineral product in an herbal base. I ran out of this product while I was there and could not find the right replacements. The week before we returned, my tooth was loose again. After I arrived home and purchased my supplement, the tooth was all right again in only a few days. This incident certainly proved to me that during pregnancy one requires great nutritional vigilance. No matter how healthy my diet was, I needed additional nutrients throughout my pregnancy and vitamin supplements provided them effectively. Be sure to consult your doctor before taking any vitamin/mineral products.

Personal Observations

I felt best on the days when I ate only fruit and salads and steamed vegetables.

Animal protein is harder on your body
and leaves more waste products in your system
but it can be very tempting during pregnancy.

I drank plenty of fluids, mainly fresh orange juice and water. I shopped weekly at the local farmer's market where I bought an average of forty pounds of oranges and made juice from them. I was so fond of fresh orange juice during my pregnancy that I could not get enough of it. A diet of mostly raw fruits and vegetables gives you a light, energetic feeling. If you add some raw, unsalted seeds and nuts to this base, you will supply your body with all the nutrients it needs. This is how I eat all the time when I am not pregnant.

When I was pregnant, however, I craved more protein and starchy foods. It is best to stick to whole grains and their products for starches. Nuts, seeds and soy products will provide you with extra protein. Animal protein is harder on your body and leaves more waste products in your system but it can be very tempting during pregnancy. I also find it is easier to control my weight when I do not consume animal products. The salt in animal products, plus the fact that they are so concentrated in protein and extremely hard to digest, may have something to do with this.

When it comes to keeping my weight down, salt has always caused me problems. Salt bloats me up and causes water retention, consequently adding overall weight to my body.

Resuming Normal Diet After Binging

On our flight back to America from our Norwegian vacation, I felt very unhealthy and fat. This was, after all, only a day after the sausage debacle mentioned earlier. During my last week in Norway, almost eight months pregnant, I ate everything in sight because I knew it would be a long time before I tasted my favorite childhood foods again. On the long flight, we flew first class and had many food selections. I decided to indulge myself just a little longer and figured it would not make me feel or look much worse.

When we landed in Los Angeles, my feet and ankles were swollen to twice their normal size. I was embarrassed and kept completely covered up for three days. I worried that my body would never look sexy again. It was totally swollen and I had gained six pounds in only one week of deviation from my healthy diet.

I spent the first three days back home in bed with my legs elevated to reverse the swelling in my feet and ankles. My head ached and I had dizzy spells. I was extremely irritable, much more so than when I had left for Norway, and to top it off I felt depressed. I deeply regretted going off my diet and finding out the hard way how ordinary foods affected me.

I started to restore myself with three quarts of purified water, fresh fruit juices, and fresh vegetable juices. I made "energy soup" with avocado,

I recommend shopping at a health food store where you can buy all organically grown food.

raw greens, sprouts, tomatoes, cucumber and lemons. I did not eat so much as a trace of salt, sugar, flour or animal products. I drank my nutty "milkshakes" and sweetened them with plenty of dried fruit. I also started chewing wheat grass and drinking the juice. This seemed to help heal my occasionally swollen, bleeding gums and helped to cleanse my body of toxins. After three days of cleansing, I added my vitamin/mineral supplement again and took daily walks.

After a week of this strict but nutritious cleansing program, my body and mind returned to normal. I felt happy and healthy, and I had regained my feeling of "lightness," despite the increasing weight of my pregnancy. I lost the six pounds of weight I gained during my last week in Norway but believe I added another "healthy" pound.

General Impressions of Pregnancy

Only two weeks before I gave birth, my total weight gain had been only fifteen pounds. I gained another two pounds before my baby was born, and it all seemed to be on the front of my abdomen. It looked like I was carrying a large watermelon. Except for my breasts, which had increased in size steadily during my pregnancy, the rest of my body looked exactly the same as before. I had an easy and joyous pregnancy. The small problem with my tooth and the consequences of my "wild" gourmet week in Norway were the only exceptions. I wish everyone a pregnancy as easy and healthy and happy as mine!

My Pregnancy Diet Tips

I recommend shopping at a health food store where you can buy all organically grown food.

Daily

2 quarts purified water to 2 quarts fresh orange juice: (occasionally substitute apple juice) pint fresh vegetable juice (beet, carrot, parsley, celery).

tablets vitamin/mineral supplement: (consult your doctor) Supplement should include vitamin C and water soluble vitamin E oil (400 units).

alfalfa tablets, brewer's yeast, and fresh wheat germ: Recommended in small quantities, but not every day.

sunshine: For better assimilation of nutrients, and for better well-being!

Pregnancy is not the time for an unconditioned woman to begin a program of strenuous exercise or diet modification.

herb teas: Peppermint, spearmint, chamomile, raspberry leaf, thistle.

smoothies: Frozen whole bananas/fresh fruit juices, strawberries, peaches, nectarines, plums and other fruits as available seasonally.

sorbets: Blend frozen fruits with a little water, or process through a Champion juicer.

banana manna: Frozen bananas/unsalted nuts and seeds processed through a Champion juicer.

fruit "pies": Make a crust of ground nuts/seeds and fill with mashed fresh fruits.

seed/nut "milkshakes": Blend seeds, nuts and water. Add dates and other dried fruits, carob powder for a chocolate flavor, perhaps a touch of vanilla extract.

seeds and nuts: Use only raw and unsalted types.

dried fruits: Unsulfured, preferably soaked in water overnight.

fresh fruits: Including avocado!

fresh vegetables: Alone, in salads or as "Energy Soup" including fresh mixed beans and sprouts. Green leafy vegetables are especially effective in cleansing and strengthening the entire body.

cooked vegetables: Steamed, baked or sautéed, including potatoes and yams. Use unrefined vegetable oils, raw/unsalted butter, herbal seasoning, or a touch of kelp or dulse to give them more flavor.

beans/grains: Combine beans with grains, rice, corn or seeds to form a complete protein.

soya products: Tofu, wieners, burgers, cheese, ice cream, milk.

condiments: Raw apple cider vinegar, unsalted natural ketchup and mustard, Jensen's Dry Vegetable Seasoning.

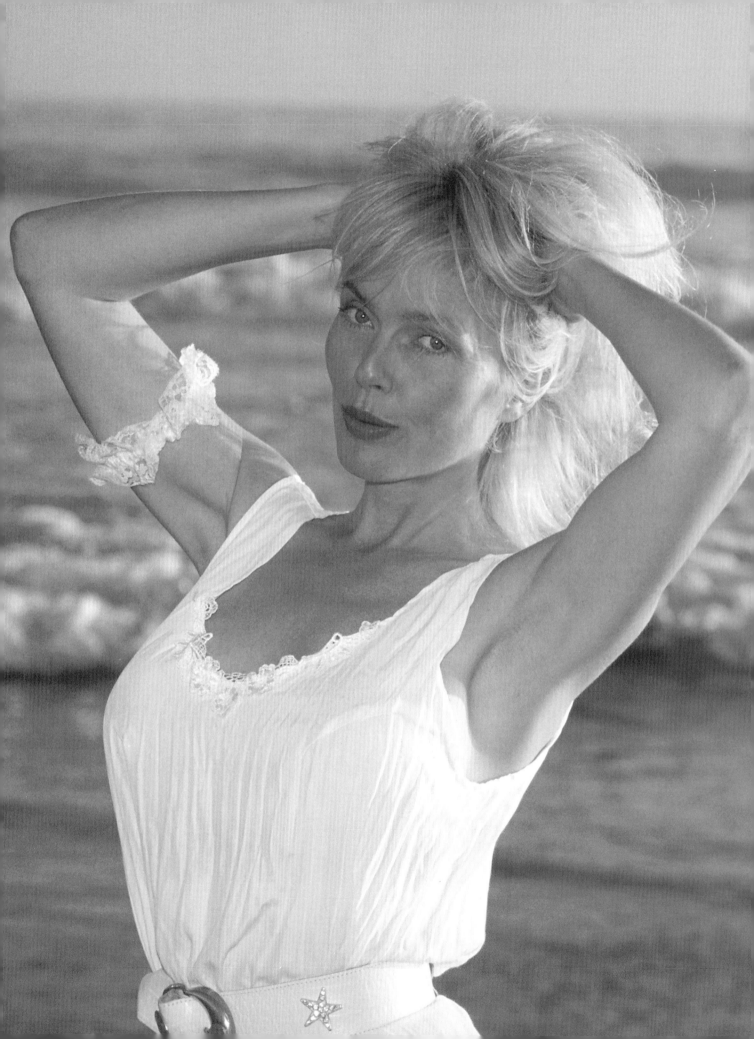

CHAPTER SIX

Holistic Awakening:
Fasting, Diets & Internal Cleansing

Your body is like a factory in which a worker can clean just one room a day and all five rooms in a week. If only one room is used each day, the cleaning will proceed without incident. If you keep that room reasonably tidy, the worker will take on additional chores. In your body's factory, jobs like eliminating toxins and burning fat can only be accomplished when the work of digestion is complete. The body will cleanse and cure itself only when it is not overtaxed by the immediate demands of digestion and elimination.

Learning to Eat Right

When I was in my early twenties, my health was not the best. I had low blood pressure, dizzy spells and endured nightly water retention in my ankles and hands. Dark circles hung under my eyes, and I was frequently depressed. No matter how much success I had in my work or how wonderfully my boyfriend treated me, life did not excite me very much. To the outside world, I had a successful career, was financially secure and was popular with both men and women. I also had a wonderful family and no obvious reason to feel bad about my life. Still, I was not very happy inside, and not very motivated to change. Nothing seemed to make me feel good anymore. I

Health is the first of all liberties,
and happiness gives us the energy which
is the basis of health.

Henri Amiel (1821 - 81) Swiss philosopher and writer

remember arriving at my voice teacher's house one morning, feeling absolutely horrible. All I really wanted to do was cry, and my teacher picked up on my raw emotional state. She felt there was not much point in trying to teach me anything that day, and instead, suggested I see a holistic doctor. While she was a very talented vocal coach, that particular direction was the single most important gift she ever shared with me.

I had reached a point where it was hard for me to do anything, let alone learn to sing! I couldn't think straight. My body felt sluggish and my energy level was virtually nonexistent. What I know now is that I was lacking the motivation, joy and vitality that are necessary components to doing anything well.

That evening, I arranged a meeting with a kind and enormously well-informed holistic doctor who helped change my way of living forever. Over the next six months, I spent two or three days each week studying with this extraordinary man and his assistant, who also happened to be his wife. I learned more about health in that time than I had previously discovered in my entire life.

The most important thing I learned was that without superior health, life was destined to be disappointing. Family, friends, money and fame can give you a great deal, but they all amount to very little without good health. What is the point of accumulating a big bankroll and many material possessions if your health is gone? Where is the enjoyment in having wonderful people in your life if you are depressed all the time? From a practical standpoint, I educated myself about the fundamental relationship between food and health. Because I was not eating well, I was not a healthy person. Because my health was so severely compromised, I was not a happy person. Your "state of body" has a very significant effect on your state of mind. A sick body is a severe impediment to sound thinking.

The key, as always, is balance, and balance cannot be attained without control of both the body and the mind. There is a great challenge in learning to eat right, cleansing your body of toxins, exercising properly, and thinking energetically. It takes both discipline and hard work to live your life to the fullest, but it is surely worth the effort! What may at first appear to be the "narrow" road will actually benefit you in the long run. I feel extremely fortunate to have learned to do what is best for myself, not what is easiest.

Holistic Awakening

After nine months under the tutelage of my holistic doctor, my body was thoroughly cleansed. As time passed, I felt better and better. With a

Natural forces
are the healers of disease.

Hippocrates (460 BC - 377 BC) Greek physician

purified body and improved health, I became a much more joyous and harmonious person. I regained the motivation to achieve my goals. I felt exuberant and was truly engaged in living my life. There is a big difference between living and merely existing, that's for sure! As you clean out your system and acquire a truly healthy lifestyle, you will understand what I am saying. This life altering change cannot be explained in words; it has to be felt!

First Step to a Healthy Lifestyle — Water!

I achieved a healthy diet by employing a number of different tactics. First, I cut out all carbonated beverages, caffeine-rich teas and milk. In other words, I gave up all the beverages I had been drinking. I substituted two to three quarts of purified/distilled water per day in addition to fresh fruit and vegetable juices. Purified/distilled water is truly the beverage of choice. Purified/distilled water is odorless and colorless and has a very fresh, clean taste which compliments all foods.

Water, Water, Everywhere!

Symptoms associated with lack of adequate water include headaches, fatigue and kidney stones. Drinking the recommended eight glasses per day is not as hard as it sounds. Make water a habit:

- *when you wake up*
- *before breakfast*
- *as you begin your morning's work*
- *late morning break*
- *before lunch*
- *late afternoon*
- *before dinner*
- *after exercise*

Foods Which Support Life

During the first nine months of my holistic program I ate only fresh fruits and salads. I also drank fruit and vegetable juices, which gave me all the vitamins and minerals I needed to stay healthy and energetic. This diet cleansed my body of the toxins which had accumulated over a lifetime of uninformed eating. For the first time in my life, I was free of the effects of animal products, grain foods, processed white flour, sugar and salt. Occasionally, when the temperature dropped and I was chilly, I ate some raw, unsalted nuts either whole or made into nut butter.

The nine months of cleansing seemed to go very quickly. I felt renewed

*A positive, joyous, constructive state of mind
will give the body tremendous energy,
whereas a negative mental attitude
will deplete your energy potential
and leave you feeling unmotivated.*

with strength and vigor. My wonderful holistic doctor often reminded me that refined sugar is a contributing factor in many diseases.

Some Thoughts About Energy

The intrinsic relationship between the psychological and physiological workings of the human body has been under examination since the seventeenth century. French philosopher René Descartes was the first to question the connection between mind and body, and scientists and philosophers have been pondering the problem ever since. Recently, scientists have discovered neurochemical substances known as endorphins in the brain, the spinal cord, glands and other body tissues. Endorphins are released during exercise and can have a pain-relieving or pleasure-inducing effect. So while the philosophical debate over the mind/body connection continues, we have scientific evidence that the body produces mood-altering substances that can have a profound effect on our energy.

A positive, joyous, constructive state of mind will give the body tremendous energy, whereas a negative mental attitude will deplete your energy potential and leave you feeling unmotivated. It is when we are pessimistic that energy eludes us. And that lack of energy leads us to make unhealthy decisions, particularly about food. Too frequently we eat to feed our emotions or simply from habit. Many people who examine their eating habits discover their urge to eat occurs for the wrong reasons most of the time. Food is meant to be the fuel that provides us with the energy for living a rich, productive life. When you sit down to eat, realize you are making a choice. For every bite you take, ask yourself, "Is this going to enhance my health and provide me with energy?" If the answer is no, you might be ready to put down your fork and pick up your running shoes.

Fasting Your Way to Good Health

During the first year of cleansing and rejuvenating my body, I learned how to fast. There are people, including some doctors, who are against fasting. I have had only positive results from it. As long as you know what you are doing and understand what the body is going through, I believe fasting is one of the best ways to help you restore your body to superior health.

Most of us have spent many years of our lives eating a diet which results in toxic residue. Together with fats and mucus, this accumulation wears down the system. We must discontinue what we are doing and make an effort to clean out the waste, or suffer the consequences. The minute you stop taking in unhealthy foods and drinks, your body starts cleansing itself.

Fasting rids the body of accumulated toxins.
It is like a thorough spring cleaning,
restoring and rejuvenating your body!

You can assist this restorative process by abolishing destructive food habits. Under Mother Nature's care, your body can be cleansed of toxic waste matter and restored to excellent health without knives or patent medicines, and everything can function in harmony.

Effects of Fasting

Fasting rids the body of accumulated toxins. It is like a thorough spring cleaning, restoring and rejuvenating your body! It also works very quickly to provide you with wonderful results. When I began a purifying diet and fasted periodically, I saw many changes in myself. My skin was more clear and beautiful, and surface wrinkles disappeared. My face and body became wonderfully firm. My eyes were much brighter and very clear. A few weeks into this program, I had almost no body odor, and even after exercising, I no longer needed a deodorant. The mucus in my nose and sinuses all but disappeared, as did my troublesome earwax. I had no abdominal bloating and my body fat decreased. Water retention, usually so noticeable in my ankles and fingers, was also gone. I needed less sleep, and while I was awake, I had much more vitality and energy. My exercise endurance level also increased. Even my hair and nails grew faster. My thinking was much more focused. The PMS symptoms, which had always bothered me, were greatly diminished. There were no more premenstrual headaches, sore breasts, or bloated feeling.

I definitely started to look younger and my face developed a "refined" look. My restored joy and peace of mind contributed to this new serenity. As my face and body revived, my confidence increased. I felt renewed hope and faith in God and myself. I started to believe that anything was possible. Now, many years into my commitment to healthful living, I believe many people do not truly get older, only more unhealthy. I feel that I am living proof that a healthy lifestyle slows down the aging process.

Help with Medical Problems

Fasting has helped me heal the occasional physical problems I encountered during my years on a cleansing diet. I have sustained good health with a good diet, but there have been short periods, for various reasons, when I cheated on my regular system or became lazy in my habits. Every time that happened, I observed a physical or mental reaction. If I stumbled into eating foods containing salt or sugar or dairy products, I would experience unhappy results from water retention and bloating to acne or a cold sore on my lip. Sometimes it was swollen glands or dark circles under my eyes. From time to time, I would experience weight gain. But if you live on a diet

When you know how to take care of yourself and stay super-healthy, you are the luckiest person in the world. People with simple, clean ways of life look young and radiant, no matter what their chronological age may be.

of natural and mainly live, raw foods, you will not have a weight problem. I eat large quantities of healthy fruit, vegetables and nuts without gaining so much as a pound. However, the minute I go off my diet and eat other kinds of foods, I gain weight very quickly. Salt, sugar, animal and grain products are much heavier, more concentrated foods than the ones on my diet. Concentrated foods have low water content which contributes to weight gain. Fruits and vegetables have a high water content and actually keep you lean and beautiful. At least that's how it works for me. Try it and see for yourself!

If I stray from my regular routine, I always go back to it quickly. It's just not worth the problems that develop. I fast at least 24 hours, and often up to three days, after I have strayed from my healthy diet. Whatever physical or mental problems develop while I am off my diet clear up very quickly once I go back on it. The results are almost immediate and my unwelcome symptoms disappear.

When you know how to take care of yourself and stay super-healthy, you are the luckiest person in the world. People with simple, clean ways of life look young and radiant, no matter what their chronological age may be. My holistic doctor always reminded me, "Through understanding and living by the physical, mental and spiritual laws of life, man has the power within to maintain a long and healthy life. A healthy man will never suffer from occasional fasting or abstaining from food."

Improved Sense of Taste, Heightened Healing

I am always amazed by the way my sense of taste is enhanced after a fast. Foods that once tasted bland seem to have a stronger flavor. You do not need to add sugar or salt to your food when you adopt this way of life. Fasting will also enhance your sense of sight, hearing, touch and smell. After a few days of fasting, your breath will be much sweeter and any bad taste in your mouth will disappear. Fasting also dissipates feelings of acid burning, indigestion and gas in your stomach. Fasting cleanses your blood and is great for your circulation. You will feel almost like a new person after you have gone through this purification program.

Eliminating Toxins

Warning: Many people opting for a water fast experience very severe elimination symptoms. In some cases, the wastes are eliminated so quickly that the result can be fatal! A person who is ill should never attempt a water fast. There are many less stressful fasts that will help you attain your goal of purification.

If you are not very familiar with the fasting process I do not recommend that you try it without qualified supervision. Fasting can be dangerous if you do not understand how it works.

If you are not very familiar with the fasting process I do not recommend that you try it without qualified supervision. Fasting can be dangerous if you do not understand how it works. Also, if you are ill in any way, do not attempt to fast without qualified supervision from a health-care specialist knowledgeable about the rigors of fasting.

There are many factors which determine how well you will feel after, as well as during, the fast. A person who has maintained an unhealthy lifestyle will experience more bad effects during a fast, as a general rule, than someone who has been on a less harmful diet all her life. The cleaner you are, the easier it is to fast and the longer you can healthily sustain it.

During the fast, the signs that toxins are being eliminated from your body are dizziness, headaches, stuffy nose, chills, aches, boils, nausea, insomnia or restless sleep and bad dreams. These reactions are collectively called a "healing crisis." They are cleansing cycles that your body must pass through on its way to restored health. Even though you are "fasting," you can speed this healing process up or slow it down. You can speed them up or slow them down according to what you eat and drink. A diet of water, fruit and vegetable juices, or raw fruit and vegetables will accelerate the process and make these symptoms more severe. A fasting diet of cooked fruits and vegetables with nuts will slow them down. This is explained in detail further below.

I cannot recommend a strict water fast of longer than a day's duration for anyone. It is much less shocking to your system to cleanse itself with fruit and vegetable juices that have been diluted by 50% with water.

Guidelines for an Extended Juice Fast
Do not attempt an extended fast without medical supervision!

For an extended juice fast, prepare diluted juices fresh every day and drink only those juices on the first day of the first week. The rest of the week, you can supplement the juice with several small meals of raw fruits and starchless, leafy-green vegetables. This enables your body to eliminate its toxins, mucus and fat at a slower rate and is less of a shock to your system.

If this type of cleansing still seems too drastic, or your body cannot handle this speed of elimination, you can further slow the process by eating heavier, more concentrated foods. Cooked starchy vegetables like corn, potatoes and yams fall into this category, as does toasted whole grain bread. When you toast or bake starchy foods, they lose many of their mucus-producing qualities. Ripe bananas are also very good when you want to slow down elimination.

Give your body a clean bloodstream
and it will function harmoniously
all your life.

On the second week of an extended fast, drink only water and diluted juices for the first two days of that week and continue to eat other foods mentioned above for the balance of the week. During the third week, have water and juices three days, and the fourth week four days, and so on, until you are drinking water and diluted juices exclusively all week. This way you build your strength up slowly. If you continue this regimen for one month, you will eliminate a lot of accumulated waste. Afterward, you can continue your healthy habit of eating fruits, vegetables and nuts with a few whole grain foods and legumes. I believe this is the best way to cleanse, build and maintain superior health.

Once or twice a year, treat yourself to a week-long cleansing juice fast. You will feel and look wonderful all your life. This way of eating and drinking is not just a diet, but a way of life. When you stray from this plan and eat unhealthy foods, don't waste your time feeling guilty. You'll recover easily by taking an extra day of the week to drink only water and juices, or eat only fruit.

No Breakfast, No Junk Foods

If a 24-hour water and juice fast is too radical a departure from your diet, start by eliminating breakfast, or eating only fruit in the morning. This is a good way to begin a fasting and cleansing program. You might experience some unpleasant sensations, such as headaches, for the first couple of days, but after that you will feel better. You will be able to work better and enjoy the other meals of your day even more. Many health problems have been cured by the "no-breakfast fast," even where the rest of the diet did not change much at all. Contrary to popular thinking, eating a "big breakfast" is not necessarily the best idea. I never eat breakfast; I only drink water and fresh juices. My lunch usually consists of fruit and nuts, and my dinner is vegetables and nuts. I drink fresh juices before each meal, and lots of puri-fied/distilled water between meals. This way I receive all the nutrients and liquids I need to maintain perfect health.

If I indulge myself in "junk food," the gratification is never worth the lack of vitality I experience the next day. I know I prolong my life and avoid disease when I continually supply my body with fruits (raw or cooked), nuts and green-leaf vegetables. There is a real payoff to maintaining an exclusive relationship with these wonderful, natural foods. Give your body a clean bloodstream and it will function harmoniously all your life.

Alternatives

If you do not like fasting on water and juices, or you find this method too

Colon cleansing is an adjunct to a healthy
lifestyle and can be discontinued
as diet and exercise improve.

extreme, there is another option. Choose an occasional day to limit your eating exclusively to one kind of fruit. This is called the "mono diet." You can also replace one of your daily meals with a mono-meal of fresh fruit. You could, for example, make one meal a day your mono-meal and do that for as long as you want. This will help your body eliminate toxins and give your digestive system a break, as fruit is the easiest of all foods to digest. Another tactic I've tried is to go on a fruit diet for a week. I call this a "camouflaged fast." It is not as drastic as drinking only water and juices, but it will cleanse and rejuvenate your system.

The Eyes Are the Mirror of More Than the Soul

Iridology is the science of analyzing the iris of the eye to diagnose the condition of your internal organs and your general health. For many years, traditional medicine has looked to the overall health of the eye as a diagnostic tool, but has ignored the significance of the iris. Today, it is possible to find doctors in the United States, Germany, Australia and the UK who support the study of the iris as an efficient health indicator.

It is important to understand that iridology reflects the causes and not the symptoms of disease. For example, the definitive diagnosis of pneumonia cannot be proved through study of the iris, but inflammation of the lungs will be discernible. A good iridologist views the iris as a mirror of your internal organs. He can tell you where toxins have accumulated in your organs or if other problems have developed in your body.

The most basic iris chart is divided into twelve radial sections like a clock face, each section corresponding to a part of the body. The iridologist assesses the basic structure of the iris and then looks for specific structural markings to show the body's strengths and weaknesses.

Internal Cleansing

No discussion of health and the benefits of cleansing is complete without discussion of cleansing the body's internal organs. All fresh fruit and vegetable juices cleanse the liver as well as the rest of your body. Drinking six to eight large glasses of purified/distilled water each day cleanses the kidneys. The fluid carries away the toxins and purifies the system. The colon can be cleansed with enemas and colonic irrigations. This cleansing often helps people who have eaten processed foods for much of their lifetime. Colon cleansing is an adjunct to a healthy lifestyle and can be discontinued as diet and exercise improve.

Enemas, on at least a weekly basis, are a very important part of my cleansing program. I feel they eliminate toxins from my body. There are divergent

Each time you remove the "garbage"
in your colon, you make room for the natural
flora to multiply.

opinions on the subject of enemas, with as many for it as against it. I believe most of the objections to enemas and colonic irrigation are from those with little or no experience with this method of natural detoxification. I can speak only for myself and tell you about my own extremely positive experience.

Colon Controversies

Some say that enemas wash out beneficial intestinal flora and valuable nutrients, and that the process is habit-forming. Others say that the purification of the large intestine and the resulting loss of harmful bacteria encourages beneficial flora to flourish. The large intestine is the only part of the colon affected by enemas. Rather than stripping the large intestine of its natural properties, proponents of this cleansing process argue that a clean environment is the best option. That is why the intestines of a newborn baby immediately begin to grow beneficial intestinal flora. Each time you remove the "garbage" in your colon, you make room for the natural flora to multiply.

The intestines are like muscular tubes with nerve endings that normally trigger peristaltic contractions when food is present. Putrefaction in the colon makes it become stagnant and weak. Each time you fill the intestines with water, however, you cause the muscles and nerves to contract with renewed vigor. It is believed that the more enemas and colon irrigations you undertake, the stronger and livelier your intestines will become. Like an arm or leg which has not been exercised, your colon can become flabby and weak. It is dependent on both exercise and cleanliness. Enemas and colon irrigation are two ways to correct conditions of filth and stagnation.

Many of us who actively participate in healthy lifestyles have heard tales of remarkable renewal associated with colonic cleansing and enemas. I have heard of one woman who had been diagnosed with a fatal illness. For two full years, she turned to a natural fruit and vegetable diet program, plus daily enemas or colonic irrigations. Her illness subsided and she achieved the vibrant, natural health which made it possible for her to work like a human dynamo for another thirty years! I would never suggest that any element of my lifestyle is a substitute for appropriate medical attention, but I do believe that my cleansing program helps me to live without need of frequent medication or visits to the doctor.

Personal Adaptation to Natural Health Practices

If the elimination organs are not functioning perfectly, the body soon becomes choked with decomposing substances much the way clogged pipes can ruin the intended function of a plumbing system. Washing deteriorating

*Many people experience only mild headaches
or a sluggish, tired feeling as warning symptoms
for months or even years before a serious
breakdown occurs in their health.*

waste from the intestines is the quickest way known to begin detoxification, and can be the first step to natural health. Elimination and assimilation are two basic cornerstones of natural health. Typically, this is a slow process. It is believed by many natural health practitioners that various waste toxins build up over a period of years to produce arthritis, ulcers, cancer, diabetes, hypertension, heart attack, stroke, etc. Many people experience only mild headaches or a sluggish, tired feeling as warning symptoms for months or even years before a serious breakdown occurs in their health.

Refined flours, sugars, chocolate confections, pasteurized milk and cheese, oily and greasy foods, cookies, cakes, etc. have long been acceptable substances in the average American diet. Most people feed on "garbage" foods and have colons with abnormal pockets, bulges and twists. Coupled with a sedentary lifestyle, elimination has become a frequent problem in today's world. Very few people have what can be considered a healthy colon. Each crooked area along the intestinal tract harbors impacted, cement-like waste deposits which adhere to the colon wall. Often these areas serve as nesting places for various parasites and harmful bacteria, and periodically, food waste forces itself through. Thus, a person can experience constipation even though his bowel movements occur two or three times daily.

Consider, as an alternative, the natural elimination which should be part of our natural health. The human body is supposed to completely evacuate the lower bowel between two and three times daily, primarily after meals. A complete evacuation should not be confused with the smaller, partial eliminations which most experience. Partial elimination does not leave the same feeling of freedom, energy and vibrant well-being. Some of the information in this section was provided by Terrence Sullivan of the Natural Health Clinic of Los Angeles.

Home Enema Program

How do you begin a home enema program? Do not eat solid foods for five hours before a colon treatment. For best results, cease eating solid foods the day before. You want to clean out what has been deposited for a long time, not what you just ate. You'll need a good enema bag, preferably the two-quart size. Fill the bag with lukewarm, distilled water, occasionally adding one teaspoon of fresh lemon juice. Hang the enema bag on the bathroom door or wall.

Apply pure olive oil or coconut oil as a lubricant, and start the enema from a position on hands and knees on the floor. As the water begins to flow in, breathe deeply to help relax the intestines and promote the free entry of water. When you feel that you cannot hold more, move to the toilet and

Get your body moving.

expel. Repeat the process until you have used the entire two quarts of water. Regular cleansing in this manner should take only five to ten minutes.

While eliminating, massage your abdominal area, do deep breathing exercises and relax. Massaging the abdomen in circular motions puts gentle pressure on the intestinal wall and loosens waste that is stuck there. Relaxation is a very important aspect of your colon treatment.

After completion of each colon treatment, take acidophilus in a goat's milk base, rejuvelac or Biotta juice containing whey. Any one of these products will help to replace the natural, beneficial bacteria in your colon. After completion, eat a nutritious meal.

Relief of Constipation or Diarrhea

Drink a pint of hot or cold water on an empty stomach as the first thing you do every morning. Peristalsis, the alternating contraction and dilation of the bowels, is strengthened when you increase bulk in your diet with lots of raw fruits, salads, nuts and seeds, sprouted legumes and grains.

If you experience loose bowels or dysentery, consume two tablespoons of carob powder (preferably raw) once or twice daily. Mix it with a little water or with a serving of nut "milk" or soy milk. Don't be overly anxious if you experience symptoms of diarrhea when you first change your diet to include more fruits and salads. Mild diarrhea is quite normal in this situation and helps to detoxify the system.

Purified/distilled water, drunk regularly, is an excellent safeguard against constipation. If you do become constipated, reach into the refrigerator before turning to the medicine cabinet. Prune juice works wonders, as do prunes soaked overnight in water or fruit juice. A tablespoon of blackstrap molasses in a glass of water before breakfast is also very helpful. Raw beets shredded into your salad will help you to remain regular and will act as a liver detoxifier as well. Most important, get your body moving. Constipation is an occupational hazard for all couch potatoes.

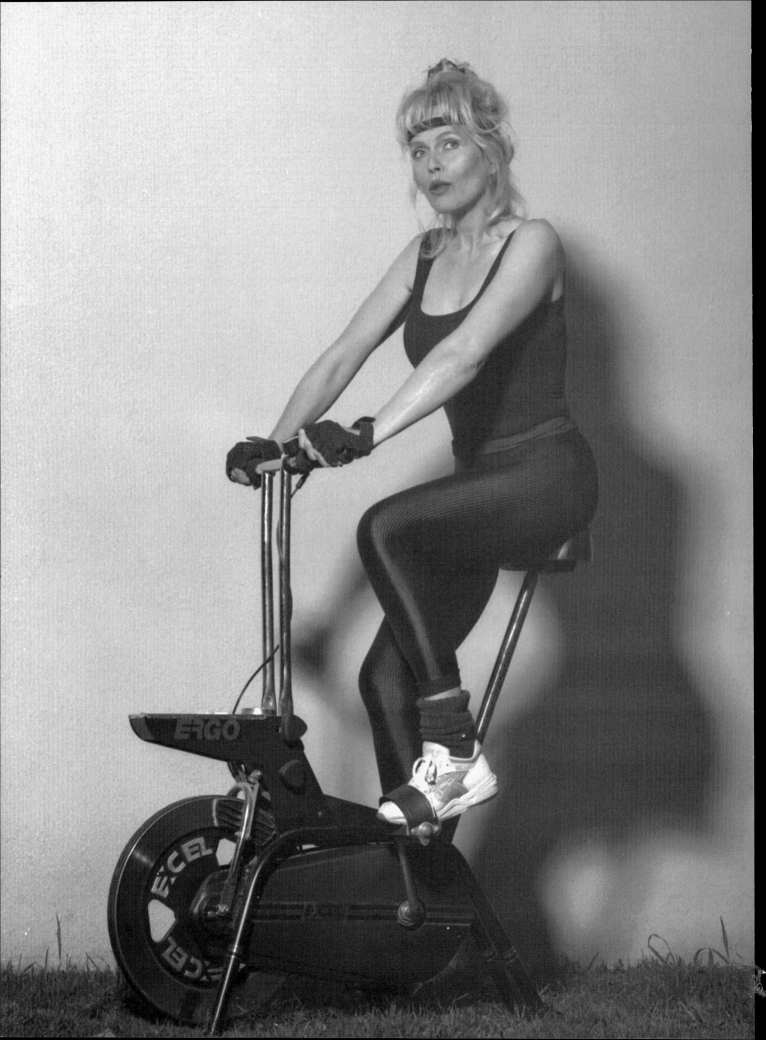

CHAPTER SEVEN

The Importance of Exercise and Fitness

Regular exercise (since my teens) has helped me stay fit, happy and successful. Without it, I fear I would be fat, unhappy and unsuccessful. Exercise has kept my body young and healthy and it has done wonders for my mental attitude. Often, when I am depressed or "down," I exercise. After a while, my dark mood vanishes.

Exercise Revitalizes

When I feel tired, I sometimes exercise instead of going to bed right away. This energizes me and motivates me to complete whatever task I had scheduled that day. If I resist feeling tired and manage to exercise, the inevitable result is one of physical refreshment and pride in my accomplishment. Exercise has done wonderful things for my self-esteem. My body has totally changed for the better. Instead of growing older and less fit, I feel I have actually become younger and more fit over the last fifteen years.

It is often hard to get started, but I make every effort to motivate myself. The rewards are always wonderful. You like yourself better when you feel good about your body. It affects your thinking in a positive way and makes you a happier, more harmonious, giving person. When you enjoy

Patients should have rest, food, fresh air, and exercise—the quadrangle of health.

William Osler (1849 - 1919) Canadian physician

yourself, you are more likely to enjoy others. When you are fit and strong in body and mind, it is easier to be the best you can be. You feel able to go out in the world, become successful, and make a difference. You can set an example and inspire others. My goal was to become a model and actress, and guarding my physical appearance had to be a priority.

I was a late bloomer. After high school, I traveled to Oslo to participate in the Miss Norway contest. It was then that I became interested in health and exercise. I found several books to study, and armed with youthful ambition and newly found information, I started toning and shaping my body. From then on, my life was never the same, and exercise became a big part of my life. My confidence slowly increased, both physically and mentally. Gone was the clumsy, insecure child I had been; the little girl who was intimidated by every other female with a nice body. Exercise and a better diet transformed me!

It is important to find an exercise you really enjoy, or combine a few favorites, and get into the habit of doing them regularly. The more you exercise, the easier it becomes. As your body starts looking better, you develop better endurance and strength, and the work becomes fun! It is virtually impossible to be really healthy without setting aside adequate time for exercise. Just as we make time for our meals and allow for sleep each night, so we must take time out for exercise. If we neglect to do so, we are bound to suffer harsh consequences.

Exercise: A Daily Routine

Exercise activates the lymphatic fluids needed to break up accumulated wastes around cells. A small trampoline, a jump rope, or even walking are helpful in this respect. Gentle bouncing for about ten minutes daily will enable the lymphatic fluids to wash back and forth over the cells, loosening waste residues so that they can be carried away in the bloodstream.

Your daily routine should also include an aerobic workout to provide muscular and cardiovascular health. Dancing, jogging, tennis, walking, swimming and weight training all fall into this category. An aerobic workout builds strength and vigor, as well as providing the stamina needed to make it through our busy days. Aerobic exercise tends to inhibit the development of osteoporosis by causing the skeletal system to absorb additional calcium. In the case of a relatively fit person, this calcium absorption compensates for the stress to which the bones are subjected. Vigorous exercise is an excellent stress reducer and enhances your energy level. Before I exercise in the morning, I drink one quart of water. As exercise enhances my blood flow, it feels like I am having an internal bath. After my exercise, I drink another quart of water. Purified water is one of the world's greatest beauty aids.

*Those who think they have not time
for bodily exercise will sooner or later
have to find time for illness.*

Edward Stanley (1826 - 93) Earl of Derby

My Personal Exercise Routine

I work out 3 or 4 days a week in the gym and 1 or 2 days at home. While I occasionally take some time off, I have found that I feel my best when I honor my commitment to my exercise program. A week or two out of the gym and I feel the negative results in both mind and body!

My Workout in the Gym

Day 1: chest—5 minutes The Bench Press machine and crossover pullies (cables)

back—15 minutes Peck Deck machine, pulldown cables for front and back, pullovers

abs—15 minutes Slantboard, slight angle

Day 2: quads (front of thighs)—15 minutes Leg Extension machine

hamstrings (back of thighs)—10 minutes Leg Curls machine and dead lifts with barbells

lower back—10 minutes Hypertension bench

calves—5 minutes Calf machine

Day 3: shoulders—15 minutes Incline Bench machine

arms—15 minutes Triceps machine

abs—15 minutes Slantboard

Day 4: quads—15 minutes Leg Extensions

hamstrings—10 minutes Dead Lifts and Leg Curls

lower back—10 minutes Hypertension bench

calves—5 minutes Calf machine

My Workout at Home

Exercycle: 30 - 60 minutes

or stair climbing: 30 - 45 minutes

lunges: (for thighs and rear end)—10 - 15 minutes

leg lifts and sit ups (for abs)—15 - 20 minutes

twists holding long stick (waist) 10 minutes

head and neck rolls (flexibility and relaxation)—3 - 5 minutes

The best way to improve circulation,
and consequently eliminate congestion,
is to maintain a daily exercise program.

I do not want too much upper body development and my routine reflects that goal. I emphasize my leg and lower body workout. To keep firm and trim but not build too much muscle, I do 15 reps per set with low weights and keep the number of sets fairly high with minimum rests between. I work at a good pace and have the weights firmly in my control at all times. I would suggest that you consult with a personal trainer at your gym to come up with an individualized routine.

Exercise Benefits Circulation

Your body is composed of about one hundred trillion cells. The health of your body is reflected in the health of these individual cells. The bloodstream is the route through which each cell receives nourishment and throws off waste. When you exercise, life-giving oxygen is supplied to the bloodstream. Conversely, lack of exercise is responsible for systemic congestion and accumulation of wastes around your cells. Conditions of stagnation and congestion are prime contributors to most degenerative physical problems. The best way to improve circulation, and consequently eliminate this congestion, is to maintain a daily exercise program.

A Smoggy Day...

Bikers and joggers beware. Summer heat brings summer smog to much of the United States. Ozone, a component of smog, causes shortness of breath and chest tightening even when present in low levels. So what's the solution? When you're cycling for fun, hit the road very early in the day before the ozone levels peak. If you're going to be out in the high traffic, high heat of the day, you'll get some relief by using a white cotton surgical mask, available at most drugstores.

Auxiliary Benefits of Exercise

Anyone who exercises regularly describes a high or a feeling of well-being. They'll say they feel light, and you can see that they're glowing with superior health. Exercise keeps you physically and mentally alert. People with regular exercise programs talk about an ability to remain focused when their non-exercising co-workers tire out. Exercise gives you pep, but allows you to feel relaxed. There is no doubt that exercise is the perfect sleep aid. Exercise is a crucial component in any weight loss plan. There is very little excess fat on a

There is very little excess fat on a body
that is regularly exercised, no matter its age.
Exercise improves blood circulation
and strengthens heart action.

body that is regularly exercised, no matter its age. Exercise improves blood circulation and strengthens heart action. It can make you look years younger and slow down the deterioration that comes with age. Exercise helps you eliminate lactic acids and other waste products which may fatigue your body. Proper exercise and good circulation ensure proper elimination of wastes from the body. If you've grown used to a sedentary lifestyle, you'll need to summon a great deal of will to walk those extra blocks to work, or swim for 30 minutes each morning. But I promise you, a lifelong commitment to exercise will become the biggest habit you'll never want to break.

What Works for You?

EXERCISE	WORKOUT	BENEFITS
swimming	cardiopulmonary stamina, chest, arms, upper back	Water provides a full-body, particularly stress-free workout for joints. Calming environment, great for beginners.
cycling	cardiovascular system, lower body, thighs, calves	Pleasant group activity, minimizes muscular pounding.
aerobic class or tape	all muscle groups, cardiovascular stamina	Group or solitary activity, great variety possible.
weight lifting	all muscle groups	Opportunity to isolate muscle group for superior toning.
walking	cardiovascular system, lower body-calves, hamstrings, buttocks, stomach	Easy access. Easily monitored workout for beginners.

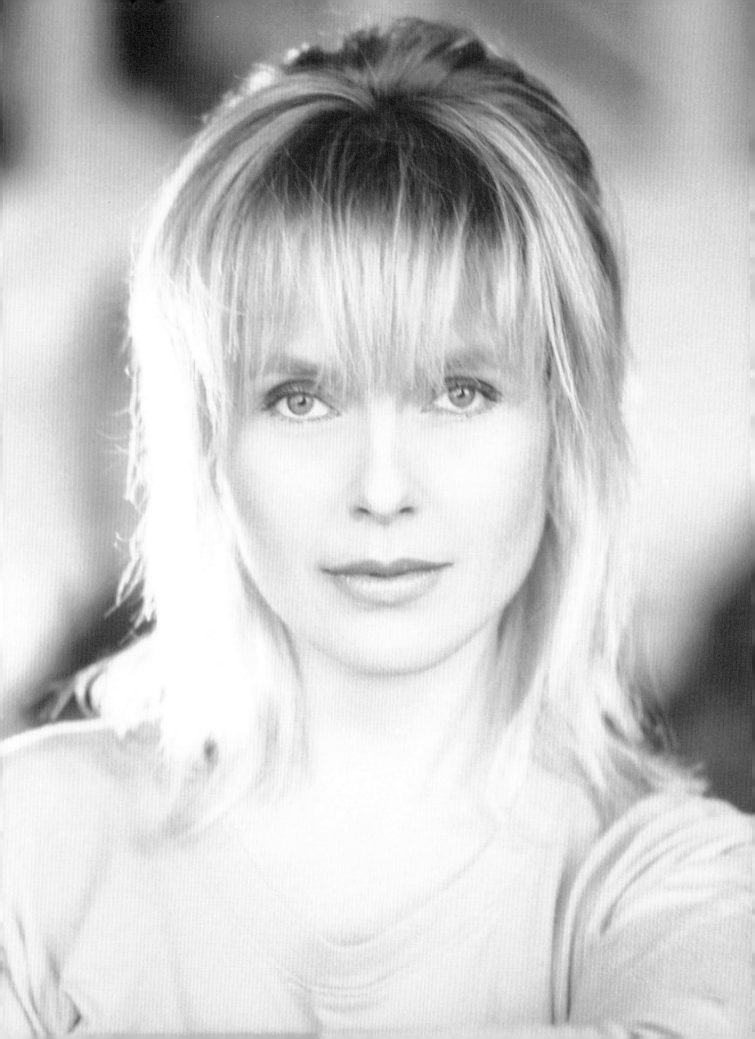

CHAPTER EIGHT

Timeless Beauty Tips

Beauty is most successfully attained through natural means. We have all seen women who attempt to camouflage the ravages of unhealthy living with heavily applied make-up. In truth, there is no substitute for the bright eyes and clear skin that are a natural dividend of healthy living. As with personalizing your exercise and nutritional programs, you will want to customize a beauty routine that works for the demands of your lifestyle. I hope you will choose those elements of my beauty routine that work for you.

A Simple Meditation to Begin Your Day

A relaxed, appreciative state of mind is an important part of any beauty regimen. I like to spend at least a few moments each morning meditating on happy things in my life; the many simple pleasures for which I am grateful. Begin with some breathing exercises for about five minutes each morning. Think of your lungs as balloons which inflate from the bottom upward. Exhale as completely as you can, using your chest muscles to press all the air

Health is the first muse,
and sleep is the condition to produce it.

Ralph Waldo Emerson (1803 - 82) US poet and essayist

from your lungs. Then inhale, and think of your breath delivering fresh oxygen and nutrients to every cell in your body. As you exhale again, imagine that all cellular waste is being released back into the bloodstream for eventual expulsion from your body.

Deep breathing supports your body's constant need for oxygen. You'll think with greater clarity and feel more centered and focused; you'll develop your lung capacity and stimulate the removal of wastes throughout your system. You can nourish your entire body when you breathe deeply and fill your lungs completely. As you cleanse your body of toxins, your whole being becomes more beautiful, including your skin, your eyes and your hair. You will experience renewed energy and vitality. Deep breathing is a very important part of my beauty process. Take five minutes each morning for this simple exercise. It is very invigorating.

Guided Imagery

Guided Imagery is a therapeutic technique that seeks to harness the healing and meditative powers of the mind. An individual creates a mental image of how to attain a goal. For example, if you have a headache, you try to visualize the source of the pain. Perhaps you see the knotted muscles as intertwined ropes glowing with heat. Next, you attempt to picture a remedy to the painful heat: perhaps an icy tumbler of water or a heavy silk scarf drenched with a cooling liquid. Imagine yourself applying the clear, cool water to the burning ropes.... Be patient. It can really work.

A Deep Breathing Exercise to End Your Day

At night, just before going to bed, stand in front of an open window or step outside to enjoy the evening air. Raise your arms and breathe shallowly with lips parted. Watch your mid-section going in and out as your diaphragm responds to your breathing. As your diaphragm supports your breathing efforts, it grows very strong. Next, count to four as you inhale. Hold the breath for a count of four and then count to eight as you slowly and evenly exhale. Soon you will achieve a very pleasurable rhythm. Your newfound strength will enable you to fill the lower lobes of the lungs with a large reserve of air. This oxygenation process is a wonderful way to prepare for a good night's sleep.

After several weeks of following this routine, your superior utilization of oxygen will most likely give you the inner sense of good health that many

Deep breathing helps every aspect
of metabolism because oxygenation is "life"
in the best and truest sense.

people have described as euphoria. As an additional bonus, your powerful diaphragmatic muscle soon will be firmed up and your belly will become flatter and stronger as the entire breathing apparatus strengthens. Learn to get into the habit and rhythm of counting as you walk and breathe. Remember, the more you practice this breathing technique, the better you will feel and the healthier you will be. Deep breathing helps every aspect of metabolism because oxygenation is "life" in the best and truest sense. Happy breathing!

Skin Care

Your skin is the largest organ of your body, and the major site for your elimination process. When you exercise and perspire, many impurities exit through the skin. The skin is cleansed by sweating, and the more you sweat, the better this process functions. Saunas, steam baths, and hot soaks in a tub have been used for thousands of years to promote better health. It is also advisable to wear natural fabrics such as cotton, to allow your skin to "breathe."

I strongly recommend that you use a dry brush to massage your skin before you shower. The combination of exercise and massage improves circulation and sloughs off dead skin cells. It is important to clean away the impurities which rise to the surface of your skin so that your skin can breathe freely. Exercise, dry brush massage and frequent showers support this process. Finish your shower with cool water to help close the pores. Your skin will look radiant and soft. You will feel great and be beautiful.

I also believe in brief sunbathing sessions on a regular basis to help eliminate toxins. Sunbathing is an excellent "invisible" waste eliminator. It rejuvenates the skin and leaves it silky with natural golden tones. It is

Skin Soothers from the Garden

Aloe vera, the thick gel obtained from the aloe vera plant, is an ideal home remedy for dry skin, sunburn and eczema. Aloe is particularly well suited to sensitive facial skin. Simply cut a section of leaf from a plant and squeeze the cooling gel onto the irritated area. Also available in bottled form at drugstores and stores that sell health products.

Calendula, also known as pot marigold, has long been a favorite among mothers. Calendula cream, available in most health food stores, can be safely applied to sore nipples resulting from breast feeding and is an excellent remedy for diaper rash, and can be used as a hand and foot cream when skin is paticularly dry.

I always say beauty
is only sin deep.

Saki (Hector Hugh Munro; 1870 - 1916) British writer

important to secure enough life-giving fresh air and sunshine, so essential to health and happiness. The direct rays of the sun on the naked body supply a type of electricity, energy and vitality to what has been called the "human storage battery." It is essential to feel the renewed vigor and strength which comes from this source.

For a Good Day, Try Sunshine

Experts recommend that if you want to sunbathe, up to 30 minutes of sun exposure with sunscreen is beneficial before 10:30 a.m. or after 2:30 p.m.

It is important to apply a good sunscreen to your face and body if you have light skin and are sensitive to the sun. Look for a brand that is swim- and sweatproof, and reapply it frequently.

Dry Brushing Skin Care

I usually spend five minutes dry brushing my skin. This is a wonderful treatment and significantly increases blood flow at the skin's surface. You can use a natural bristle brush, mitt or loofah. I prefer a bristle brush because its long handle enables me to reach all the way down my back.

Dry brushing enhances immune system function, assists lymphatic drainage, and aids in the elimination of the cellulite wastes lurking just below the surface of your skin. (Deep breathing also helps expel these wastes, which contribute to cellulite.) By revitalizing nerve endings in your skin, dry brushing improves skin function and provides a healthy glow. It also improves muscle tone and aids in cell renewal. Dry brushing for just five minutes each day will open your pores and cleanse your skin without removing natural oils. Brushing your skin improves overall complexion and makes you look younger and feel better. It wakes you up!

Dry Brushing Technique

A daily dry brushing routine is best undertaken before you shower. I begin by brushing my hands and fingers in any direction seven or eight times. Then I brush in long strokes, first from the wrist to the elbow, then from the elbow to the shoulder. From there, I brush forward to my heart and down my torso. I brush across the tops of my toes to the soles of my feet, and up toward my ankles. The soles of your feet are sensitive, but start out gently, and eventually you will get used to the scratchy feel of the brush. Continue by brushing the

Health is beauty, and the most perfect health
is the most perfect beauty.

William Shenstone (1714 - 63) English poet

entire surface of each leg from ankle to knee, then from knee to thigh. Always brush with light strokes, upward to the heart.

Now, gently hold the brush against your neck, vibrating the bristles in place. Next, brush your neck in downward motions, and then swing the brush gently across the top of your shoulders. To stimulate the lymphatic system, hold the brush under either armpit and rotate it back and forth several times. On the front, sides and back of your body, use long sweeping single strokes, always in the direction of your heart. To help rid yourself of any cellulite at the tops of your thighs and buttocks, brush upward with circular strokes in these areas.

Wet Cleansing

After I finish dry brushing, I take a nice warm shower and finish with an invigorating splash of cool water to close my pores. To help your skin retain the moisture it has absorbed during a bath or shower, apply a rich body lotion immediately afterward. I have had great success with body lotions containing sea moss, ivy and spearmint. Each of these ingredients plays an important role in reviving the skin and helping to control cellulite. I also look for ingredients such as canola oil, which holds moisture in but allows my skin to breathe. Remember that your body, like your face, needs daily attention to remain smooth. Use a non-drying, pH-balanced body scrub instead of soap, and apply body lotion every day. Soon you will notice a wonderful difference in your skin's texture.

Finally, I clean my face thoroughly each morning. Cleanliness is the most important variable in the pursuit of a beautiful complexion. First, I apply a natural cleanser to slough off dead skin cells on the surface and remove any traces of make-up that might be left from the night before. I always warm my hands by rubbing them together before applying the cleanser. This additional heat liquefies the cleanser, helping it to spread more readily and penetrate more effectively.

Two days a week, I use a special scrub or a steamer to deep cleanse my skin. This is the ultimate in skin care. First I apply a natural facial scrub and gently massage it into my skin with small circular motions. Sea kelp and sea salt are among the ingredients I look for in a scrub or mask. They help smooth the skin texture and have anti-bacterial qualities which help prevent skin eruptions.

For maximum effect, give yourself five minutes of steam while the scrub is still on your face. If you do not own a facial sauna appliance, use a pot of steaming hot water and a towel draped over your head to tent your face. The steam opens the pores and allows for deep cleansing. After the treatment, your

I can assure you that if you put in the time
to take care of your skin
you will be rewarded each day
when you look into the mirror.

skin will be radiant. Scrubs and masks give the skin a polished look because they remove dead cells which dull the skin giving it an uneven texture. Make sure to rinse well and remove all traces of the cleanser. Most days I go straight from cleanser to toner, bypassing the extra time it takes for a deep cleansing scrub and steam. A good natural toner closes your pores and helps keep your skin smooth and fresh. Rinse the toner from your face with cool water.

Make sure that the cotton balls you use to apply toner or remove make-up are made from 100% cotton. Synthetic cotton balls do not have the gentle, non-abrasive properties of cotton, and tissues contain fine wood fibers which over many years of use can cause damage to your skin. I also recommend cotton balls for removing nail polish.

The final step in your facial routine is moisturizing. To ensure maximum effectiveness, I apply my moisturizer while my face is still damp. The vitamins, herbs and vegetable oils in my facial moisturizer nourish and protect my skin. Vitamin E additives are particularly important. Vitamin E contains tocopherol-linoleate, which is part of the natural oil that holds skin cells together. It penetrates the skin and stays active for six to twenty hours. Moisturizers containing this form of vitamin E are the most effective aids in retaining youthful, healthy skin. Sunflower oil, evening primrose and avocado oil are also excellent items to have in your moisturizer.

Pay special attention to the areas around your eyes and on your neck. There are few oil glands in these trouble spots, and they will be the first to show the aging effects of dryness. Reapply moisturizer to these areas several times each day. Having good skin is a matter of commitment. I can assure you that if you put in the time to take care of your skin you will be rewarded each day when you look into the mirror.

The Wonders of the Slant Board

I heartily recommend five to ten minutes on the slant board twice a day for a radiant complexion and a rejuvenated attitude toward living. The opportunity to lie down with your feet elevated well above your head offers a rare reprieve from the constant forces of gravity on all your internal organs.

Warning: Not everyone is an appropriate candidate for the slant board. Pregnant women, individuals with high blood pressure, anyone who has experienced internal bleeding, people with a history of fainting or who are obese are all counseled against the use of the slant board.

*To lose a lover or even a husband or two
during the course of one's life can be vexing.
But to lose one's teeth is a catastrophe.*

Hugh Wheeler (1912 - 87) British-born US writer

Dental Hygiene

I continue my morning with about a half hour stint in the bathroom. I brush my teeth with a natural toothpaste. Sometimes I alternate the toothpaste with a mixture of salt and baking soda, which is very effective for strengthening gums, eliminating plaque and whitening teeth. My formula is one teaspoon salt, one teaspoon baking soda and a little peroxide (2%) to create a paste.

First I wipe the paste on the sides of my teeth so that it penetrates into the spaces between my back teeth. To do this, I point the bristles of my toothbrush up into the gums and wiggle. Don't brush back and forth. In time, that will cut into the sides of your teeth and may actually result in the need for a filling. When the sides of your teeth feel squeaky clean, use floss to work the paste against the front and back surface of each tooth. Use water to rinse out the salt, baking soda and dislodged plaque mixture. If your gums bleed, wipe some additional paste on the trouble spot and let it remain there for a while. When this is done correctly, the gums will become healthier, and after three or four applications, there will be no bleeding at all.

This dental care routine is very effective in eliminating plaque, which is a leading cause of bad breath and periodontal disease. To keep your mouth clean and healthy, it is also important to have regular dental checkups at least twice a year.

Magical Mystery Paste

There's really no mystery here. This winning combination works as well as numerous commercial tooth care preparations for a fraction of the cost.

Salt kills harmful bacteria and fungi by dehydration.

Baking soda changes the pH (acid/base balance) of your entire mouth, causing many harmful organisms to give up residence in hard-to-clean places between your teeth and under your gums.

Peroxide kills organisms through oxidation reactions.

Make-Up

After I have taken the time to purify my thoughts and beautify my skin, I spend only a few minutes on my make-up, applying a touch of blush to my cheeks and a light lip liner on my lips. I never use mascara, foundation, powder or eye shadow unless I'm going out for something special.

You can buy wonderful, pure products
in natural health food stores: shaving creams,
shampoos, conditioners, toothpaste, moisturizers
and body lotions, facial cleansers and toners,
deodorants, masks and scrubs
and cleansing bars—all chemical free!

In my line of work, I have had to learn the basics of make-up application in order to be well prepared for a job or an interview. First I smooth on a waterbase liquid foundation around my eyes, then down my face, with a tiny amount on my forehead. I put a touch of concealer under my eyes, especially when I have not had enough sleep.

Next I apply blush and shading tint, beginning at the hollow of my temple near the hairline and in an arc along the edge of my cheekbones. After that I apply eye shadow in a light shade to compliment my fair complexion. I use a slightly darker shade on my eyelid than under my browline. Sometimes I take a shortcut and apply the same shading tint I use on my cheeks as eye shadow. If I use an eyeliner, I draw a very fine line as close to my lashes as possible. Then I use a little mascara. Finally, I like to use both lip liner and lipstick, with just a touch of lip gloss.

Throughout the day, I apply a small amount of moisturizer to my face and hands. I might also spray my face with purified water because the air in Los Angeles is very dry. A good moisturizer is an indispensable product. I stay away from beauty products which contain strong chemicals. I want my beauty aids to be as pure as possible. You can buy wonderful, pure products in natural health food stores: shaving creams, shampoos, conditioners, toothpaste, moisturizers and body lotions, facial cleansers and toners, deodorants, masks and scrubs and cleansing bars—all chemical free!

Go for the Green!

Masks have been used for centuries to moisturize dry or mature skin. And there's the added bonus of the "slow down factor." There is not a lot of rushing around you can do when you're under the spell of the avocado.

Combine one quarter of a ripe avocado with one teaspoon of yogurt. Mix well and apply to your face and throat. Now, the best part: Put on your favorite music, lie down and relax for 20 minutes. Remove mixture with a warm washcloth.

Seaweed Bath

I try to make time each week for a warm, relaxing seaweed bath. Look for seaweed bath products in natural food stores and at some beauty salons. Seaweed has a detoxifying effect on your body and a hydrating and toning effect on your skin. While I soak, I stimulate the skin cells further with a loofah. Relaxing in a

When I think of women,
it is their hair which first comes to my mind.
The very idea of womanhood is a
storm of hair…

Friedrich Nietzsche (1844 - 1900)

tub of warm water is emotionally soothing and helps reduce stress, a major contributor to wrinkles and cellulite. Soak for 20 to 30 minutes for best results.

Relief for Aching Muscles

A warm bath is a welcome retreat if you've overdone it at the gym. For a little extra help with sore muscles, try this soothing bath salt recipe:

Into a ten inch square of muslin pour 1/2 cup of Epsom salts, 1/2 cup of baking soda, 1 tablespoon each of sage, marjoram, chamomile, pine needles, 2 teaspoons each of lemon balm and peppermint and 10 drops essential oil of eucalyptus or juniper. Gather the edges up and tie the bundle with string. Run under warm tap water for one minute. Get into warm (not hot) tub and gently massage your body with the bath salt bag for several minutes, then let the bag float in the tub while you enjoy a restful soak. Discard bath salts after use.

Hair Care

When I wash my hair, I use natural hair care products from a health food store. Pure botanical ingredients such as rosemary, nettles, chamomile and silica strengthen the hair and give it shine and luster.

My hair has a tendency to become brittle as a result of highlighting every three months. I use an oil treatment twice monthly to counteract the inevitable chemical damage to my hair. Oil treatments help restore the hair's natural elasticity and shine, making it appear fuller and healthier. I have also found massage to be greatly beneficial to the hair and scalp. I use a gentle but firm rotating motion with my fingertips to apply pure essential oils diluted with vegetable oils, such as sweet almond, jojoba or walnut. For oily scalp and hair, apply essential oils of rosemary, lavender and geranium. Several drops diluted with a small amount of vegetable oil is usually enough. Cedar wood oil, a thick resin, works well with dry hair and scalp.

After massaging the oil into my scalp, I brush my hair vigorously from the scalp to the ends with a natural boar-bristle brush to distribute the scalp oils evenly and remove any residue. This also stimulates blood flow to the scalp and opens pores, allowing oils to enter and feed the hair follicles.

For dry or chemically damaged hair, let the oils remain on overnight and wash thoroughly in the morning. Always use a rubber brush on wet hair. Style with care and use a blow dryer with multiple heat settings to prevent heat damage to your hair. Every session on the slant board is a bonus to your hair, as the blood flows freely to the scalp and stimulates hair

*Always wear a sun hat and protective clothing
to cover as much of your skin as possible
when you are out in the sun too long.*

growth. If you don't have a slant board, lie across your bed allowing your head to hang down over the edge for several minutes. Then brush out your hair for added stimulation to the scalp. Consider this a "scalp exercise" you do once a week.

Nontraditional hair salons are starting to appear in major cities. They use natural products and promote alternative treatments such as aromatherapy, hair-loss remedies, enzyme hair coloring and hair painting, herb coloring and aromatherapy perms. If your salon does not offer these natural hair care services, encourage the owner to look into them, or perhaps seek out another salon. Natural products free of harsh and damaging chemicals are growing in popularity. If you express a desire to try them, the salon owner may be convinced to try them too.

Natural Highlight Helpers

for brown or black hair —rosemary, sage, quassia chips, walnut hulls
for blonde hair —chamomile, crushed rhubarb root, fresh lemon juice
   (before sunbathing)
for red hair—calendula
Bring 3 cups of distilled water to a boil and remove from heat. Add three heaping tablespoons of the chosen herb mixture, then stir and cover. Steep for 30 minutes, and strain and store in a glass or plastic bottle. After shampooing, gently squeeze excess moisture from hair. Pour and work a generous amount of the highlighter into hair. Gently squeeze out excess, and style hair as usual. Store in fridge for up to two weeks.

Whether you go to a salon or style your hair at home, it is important to maintain strong, healthy-looking hair. During the summertime it may be particularly difficult to keep your hair from looking dull and damaged, especially if you enjoy suntanning and swimming. Wear a hat or scarf to shield your hair and scalp from the hot sun. Massage essential oils into your hair and scalp before you expose it to the sun's rays. They help protect it from damage, and heat from the sun actually helps the oils penetrate and condition your hair. (See *Delicious* Magazine, July/August 1992.)

Be Sun Smart!
Always wear a sun hat and protective clothing to cover as much of your skin as possible when you are out in the sun too long. Find sunglasses with

A sunscreen should contain moisturizing
and skin care ingredients
such as organic oils and herbs like rosemary,
yarrow and pansy; even bee pollen is beneficial.

100% UV filters to protect your eyes from ultraviolet radiation.

The sun's heat dehydrates your skin. Drink plenty of water before, during and after sun exposure to replenish lost moisture and to prevent further drying. Avoid or minimize prolonged sun exposure between 10:30 a.m. and 2:30 p.m. when UV rays are strongest and most damaging. Drinking plenty of water counteracts dry skin from within and promotes skin suppleness and elasticity. Bodies use and lose large amounts of water during hot weather, so liquid refreshments should always be kept handy.

Apply natural sunscreen to lips, ears, back of neck and tops of feet. Those are areas people usually forget to cover. A sunscreen should contain moisturizing and skin care ingredients such as organic oils and herbs like rosemary, yarrow and pansy; even bee pollen is beneficial.

I sometimes make my own sunbathing lotion by mixing half coconut oil and half pure aloe vera gel together. Aloe has a built-in sunscreen, and this combination turns my skin a beautiful golden tan without dehydration. After my sunbath, my skin feels soft and moist, but I rub on more aloe vera gel to make sure it stays that way. Aloe vera gel works well if you develop a sunburn. It feels very cool when you put it on and helps protect against permanent sun damage.

Lemons, Seaweed and Tea Tree Oil

Lemon wedges are fantastic cleansers. I use lemon on my face to banish oily patches from around my nose and chin, especially when I anticipate my period. Sometimes I use lemon to cleanse my skin before I shower. It is wonderfully refreshing. When my hands are especially dirty and there is dirt under my nails, lemon seems to work better than soap.

Seaweed is a mineral-rich vegetable from the ocean that is very beneficial for both your beauty and health. Sea plants are constantly bathed in sea water, which provides them with a rich supply of nutrients. The Japanese are famous for their creative use of seaweed as a food. Now people everywhere are eating seaweed because it is low in fat and calories and high in fiber and nutrients. These sea vegetables also protect us against cancers of the digestive tract. Marine flora possess numerous medicinal properties, including antibiotic, antiviral, anti microbial, and antifungal agents. Seaweed is beneficial in maintaining the health of the mucus membranes. It can treat some arthritic and nervous disorders, and has been credited with alleviating constipation, rheumatism, colds and skin irritations.

Travel is glamorous only

in retrospect.

Paul Theroux (b. 1941) US-born writer

When used as a body scrub, *sea kelp* and *sea salt* help smooth the skin texture. They are slightly abrasive, contain antibacterial qualities, and help clean up skin eruptions.

Tea tree oil has been called "the medicine kit in a bottle." Pure and natural tea tree oil is extracted from only one of 600 species of Australian tea tree, called *melaleuca alternifolia.* The pure, fragrant, golden oil is an excellent germicide, fungicide and antiseptic when it is used in its natural state. It performs the same functions when it is added to such products as creams, gels, shampoos and conditioners. Tea tree oil is used to control dry hair, dandruff, itchy scalp, scaly patches, fever blisters, cold sores, insect bites, acne, poison oak and ivy, earache, chapped lips and toothache pain. It is also a fine breath freshener, mouthwash and gargle and can be used as an inhalant. On the body and feet, it is applied to treat dry skin, sports injuries, insect bites, cuts and abrasions, bruises, sprains, muscle aches, herpes-like lesions, vaginal problems, itchiness, corns, calluses, ingrown toenails and nail fungus problems. Its healing, antiseptic, germicidal and astringent properties make it one of the most efficient natural beauty aids I have ever used.

Travel Tips

Travel is exhausting and we can all use some pointers on how to stay beautiful while en route for business or pleasure. First, cleanse your skin thoroughly before leaving home. After cleansing, smooth a heavy-duty moisturizer onto your face and body. This moisturizer should contain humectants such as glycerin or propylene glycol. Humectants draw moisture in. Without them, water quickly evaporates from your skin and can leave you with a tickling, tight sensation.

Never wear make-up when you travel because the pigments will dry out your skin. If you are wearing make-up, it is advisable to remove it as soon as you board the plane. Be sure to keep face and body lotion handy to use on your feet and hands.

Use natural spray mist on your face and hair before your skin starts to feel dry, but be careful not to overspray. Also, continue to apply moisturizer throughout your trip. Just before you arrive at your destination, remove any extra moisturizer, put on your make-up and style your hair. If you use gels and sprays on your hair, try non-drying alcohol-free products. In the case of an extended flight, soak cotton pads in chamomile tea and store them in a plastic bag. Placing them on your eyes will relax you and prevent puffiness. You can also put these presoaked pads under the eye masks provided by

There are no ugly women,
only lazy ones.

Helena Rubinstein (1882 - 1965)

many airlines to help passengers sleep. The only make-up I use when I travel is a blush and lip gloss. This way it is very easy to cleanse my skin and apply fresh moisturizer before I land. A touch of mascara and fresh blush and lip gloss just before touchdown make me look presentable and I feel composed on arrival. I don't have to hide behind dark glasses and a floppy hat.

To cleanse the skin and get rid of puffy eyes, alternate warm and cold water facial compresses. I soak a washcloth in warm water and apply it to my face and eyes for a few seconds, then I do the same with cold water. I repeat this about ten times. Soaking the skin softens it and loosens debris, allowing a more thorough cleansing. Remember to drink lots of fluids while traveling. I bring one half gallon of purified water and drink it periodically throughout my flight. This ensures skin hydration from within. Drinking plenty of water also helps maintain energy levels and decreases travel stress. Finally, a word to the wise: don't let travel interrupt your exercise routine. If you're going to be out of town on business and can't get to your aerobics class, make a visit to the hotel health club. If you're visiting family, have someone show you a safe place to jog. Try to follow this simple travel routine. I promise you'll reach your destination in fine form.

Minimizing Jet Lag

When recovering from jet lag, allow one day per time zone.

Traveling east is tougher on your internal clock because it pushes you ahead. When flying east, particularly if you expect to be clear-headed for a business meeting, choose an early departure time. When you're going west, fly in the evening if possible.

Adjust your watch to your destination time zone as soon as you board your flight and try to adjust your behavior accordingly. Eat and sleep in flight according to your destination time zone.

Basic Beauty Reminders

While I've gone into greater depth about the perils of unhealthy foods in the earlier chapters of this book, I must mention once more the importance of diet to lifelong beauty. To discover your beauty and maintain it, you should avoid all alcohol, drugs, cigarettes, caffeinated beverages and coffee, chemical preservatives, additives, flavorings and colorings. Canned and overcooked foods, salty and sugary treats, refined grains, and dairy and meat products also put stress on the body and lower natural resistance. A healthy

The stresses of daily life are not likely to forget where you live just because you manage to take a holiday.

diet of fresh fruits and vegetables, raw seeds and nuts, legumes and whole grains is best. You might even want to specify that these foodstuffs be organically grown. They will become a big part of your beauty regimen and way of life.

If you can live this way for one year, you will observe enormous results. You will feel great, be much happier and look more beautiful. People who have not seen you for a while will compliment you and inquire about your lifestyle. Some will even wonder if you had plastic surgery. Never underestimate the power of natural beauty!

I believe true beauty comes from within. A person who radiates joy, energy, vitality, optimism and peace cannot help but be beautiful. When you express these qualities, you exude the kind of power and charisma that cannot help but draw others to you. On many occasions, I have met people who were not picture-perfect physically, but they had so much charm and light in their eyes that I immediately perceived them as true beauties. A lack of love and joy or an overwhelmingly negative attitude can make a person unattractive and difficult to enjoy. Constructive thinking and a loving, giving, joyous soul makes people shine with beauty.

These qualities do not disappear with age. A person who has this type of appeal may age chronologically, but will remain youthful and vigorous. Others are attracted to such people because they are like bundles of energy and love. Everybody feels a deep need for positive energy and will flock around people who have it. I want to be the type of woman who possesses this kind of ageless beauty as I grow older.

A Last Word on Relaxation

You know what it is like to return from a relaxing vacation and before your tan has a chance to fade, the phone is ringing off the hook and the project deadline that seemed eons away has managed to escape you. The stresses of daily life are not likely to forget where you live just because you manage to take a holiday. Our lives are too busy to rely only upon vacation time to provide us with an opportunity to relax. I try to set aside 20-30 minutes each day for some quality relaxation time. Many people complain that they are too busy to take time out of the day to indulge in relaxation. But I know that the more hectic my schedule is, the more I need to rejuvenate myself.

First you must make the commitment to yourself that you will not be distracted. Turn the ringer off the phone. There is no need to have any sound from the radio or television. Dim the lights or turn them off. Loosen any tight clothing or jewelry. You can lie down or sit comfortably. Use pillows to

Exuberance is beauty.

William Blake (1757 - 1827) British poet

support your neck and the small of your back if you are sitting. If you choose to lie down, add a pillow under your knees to avoid any lower back pressure. Take a moment to settle into a comfortable position.

Now, with your eyes closed, breathe as you normally would and become aware of your breathing. Take a cleansing breath in through your nose and exhale through your mouth. Notice where you are holding tension in your body. Breathe again and let go of that tension as you exhale. Repeat this several times until you have grown more relaxed. Then, beginning with your toes and going up each leg, tighten individual muscle areas as you inhale and then relax the muscle as you exhale. Repeat as you move from your toes, to your calves, thighs, buttocks, back, abdomen, chest, shoulders, neck, then down to fingers, hands, arms, back to the neck, and finally to the back of your head and your face. I release the tension in my face by making exaggerated faces: opening my mouth wide, sticking out my tongue, raising my eyebrows and wrinkling up my nose. (You can see why it helps to do this alone!)

I finish with a couple of cleansing breaths and lie there for a few minutes more, slowly allowing the world to filter back into my consciousness. Finally I open my eyes, look around and slowly sit up. Believe me when I tell you that after this half hour "indulgence" I am ready to take on the world!

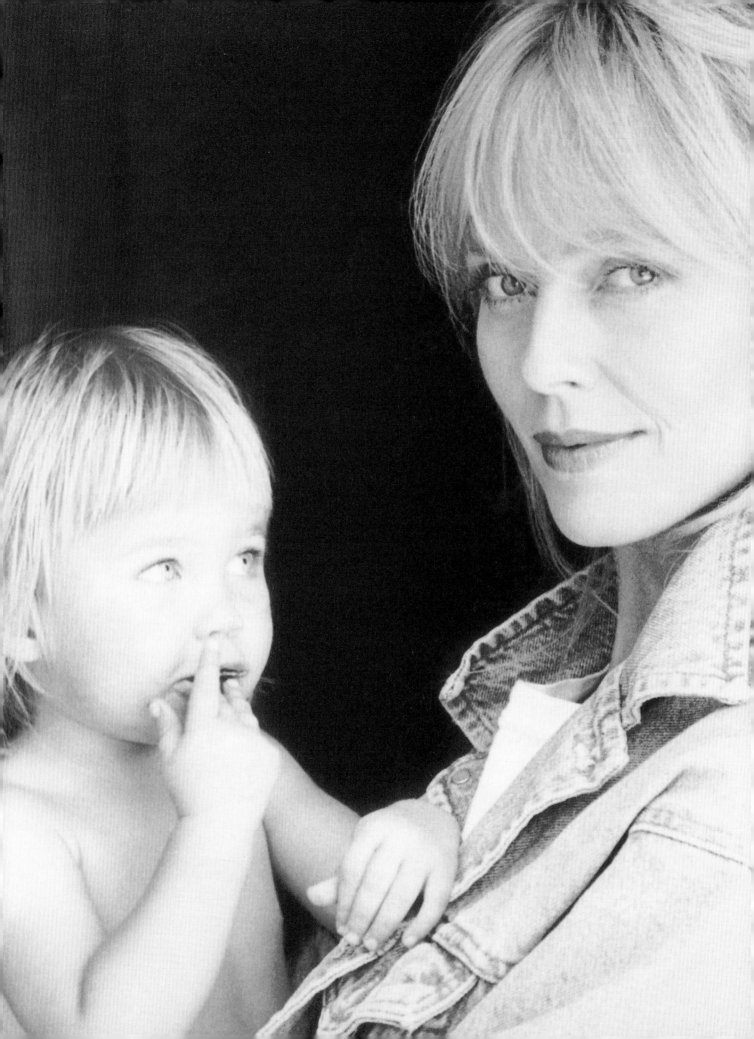

CHAPTER NINE

Aging Reversed

When I think of myself at eighty or ninety years old, I never imagine being sick, or unproductive. I feel I have the information I need to make so-called old age a very peaceful, productive and happy time. I believe at that advanced age I will have accumulated a great deal of wisdom about life, nature, people and myself. Because of all my knowledge about health and longevity, I also believe I will still have a youthful and disease-free body and will be able to enjoy life to the fullest. I imagine I will have gained much wisdom while maintaining a healthy body. Isn't that what it is all about?

Think of how much you can do in life in your ninth or tenth decade of living; how productive you will be, and how much you will be able to give back to life! There is no need to worry about getting older chronologically when you have the ability and knowledge to keep a healthy mind and body

Life begins at forty.

Sophie Tucker (1884 - 1966)

for as long as you live. Then you can really live your life to the fullest. We want to remain healthy for a lifetime, physically and mentally. Stay full of love and joy and optimism no matter what happens. Construct a good mental attitude, exercise regularly, and eat right. You will be well on your way to staying healthy forever.

Research on Aging

Free radical theory is being discussed frequently in the current literature on aging. Two researchers, Michael Murray, M.D., and Joseph Pizzorno, M.D., are simultaneously evaluating two aging theories —the programmed theory and the damage theory. The programmed theory maintains there is a genetic clock ticking away that determines when old age sets in. The damage theory contends that aging is a result of cumulative damage to cells and genetic materials.

The damage theory, sometimes called the free radical theory, is the only one that lends itself to intervention. It claims that destruction caused by free radicals, molecules that bind to and destroy cellular compounds, contributes to aging and age-related disease. Free radicals come from sunlight, X-rays, radiation and chemicals. Other sources include cigarettes; air pollution; pesticides; anesthetics; petroleum-based products; food which has been fried, barbecued or char-broiled; alcohol; coffee; and solvents found in compounds like cleaning fluids, paint and furniture polish.

Most free radicals in the body are toxic oxygen molecules. Ironically, oxygen, the element that sustains us, is also responsible for aging since it oxidizes in the body. In a way, this process can be compared to rusting. Certain people seem to deteriorate earlier than others. Compounds that prevent this type of damage are referred to as antioxidants. One of the most important aspects of nutrition and longevity now being researched is the role of antioxidants and their effect on free radicals. A large number of studies have demonstrated that dietary antioxidants can increase life expectancy. Murray and Pizzorno feel dietary antioxidants may decrease the incidence of cancer as well.

Antioxidants act like scavengers, seeking out and neutralizing free radicals. More specifically, they retard the aging process by inhibiting harmful environmental influences, reducing the oxidation of essential dietary nutrients and preventing the degenerative process initiated by free radicals.

Antioxidants and Free Radicals

For many years, research into aging has focused on free radicals. These free radicals contribute to telltale signs of aging, such as wrinkled skin, by snatching electrons from stable substances in the body. This causes the stable substance to

It takes a long time to grow young.

Pablo Picasso (1881 - 1973)

become unstable and the result is cellular damage. The body repairs damage from thousands of free radical assaults which occur every day. Through time, as a person ages, the body performs these repairs less efficiently.

Since the advancement of the free radical theory of aging, research has touted antioxidant compounds, such as vitamins A, E, C and selenium, for their successful anti-aging properties. Antioxidants seem to reverse the destructive action of free radicals and also help combat such serious conditions as cancer and heart disease. A research team discovered that men with low blood levels of vitamin C and carotene—both of which are found in brightly colored vegetables such as carrots—suffered more frequently from cancer.

And You Thought They Just Tasted Good

Food scientists are unleashing some of the most potent weapons in their arsenal to assist in the fight against cancer. The good news is that we can jump in on the winning side as well, by eating right. Scientists call these cancer-fighting substances phytochemicals.

Tomatoes: The antioxidant properties of vitamin C help the tomato to absorb dangerous free radicals.

Citrus Fruits: Limonene in oranges, lemons and other citrus fruits helps to raise levels of naturally occurring enzymes that break down carcinogens.

Broccoli and Cabbage: These are some of the big guns in the fight against cancer. Indoles, present here as well as in Brussels sprouts, cauliflower and bok choy, affect estrogen metabolism, prompting the body to create hormones that discourage the growth of cancerous breast tissue.

Garlic and Onions: Allium compounds in the onion family increase levels of enzymes thought to break down substances before they become carcinogenic. And the boost to the immune system doesn't hurt!

Specific Antioxidant Compounds

Since antioxidants have been shown to slow down the aging process, I want to mention the most potent anti-aging agents below and tell you a little about how they work.

Vitamin C: Many clinical, experimental and population studies have shown that increased vitamin C intake yields many beneficial effects, including

Drink fresh carrot and vegetable juices.
They could save your life!

stronger immunity, increased life expectancy, lower cancer rates, and better ability to heal wounds.

Vitamin E and Selenium: These two antioxidants work together. If you are deficient in either one, you put yourself at higher risk of developing cancer, cardiovascular disease and inflammatory diseases. They are of extreme importance in preventing free radical damage to cellular membranes.

Zinc: Zinc helps rid the body of toxic carbon dioxide and is essential for bone formation. Normal growth and development of the sex organs and proper functioning of the prostate gland are also linked to sufficient levels of zinc intake.

Carotene: Consumption of foods rich in carotene, such as green-leaf vegetables, carrots, yams and sweet potatoes, is the best method to increase tissue carotinoid levels. For most people, carotene means vitamin A, but only thirty to fifty of more than four hundred carotinoids are believed to have vitamin A activity. Research has focused mostly on beta-carotene, but other carotenes are stronger in antioxidant activity and are deposited in tissues to a greater degree. Drink fresh carrot and vegetable juices. They could save your life!

Sulfur-Containing Amino Acids: Studies suggest that maintaining optimum levels of methionine and cysteine may promote longevity in humans. As you become older, the level of amino acids in the body decreases. The best food sources for methionine and cysteine are nuts, brewer's yeast, beans, eggs and fish.

Bioflavonoids: Bioflavonoids are a group of plant pigments which provide us with remarkable protection against free radical damage. Bioflavonoid molecules are unique in their antioxidant properties and their ability to scavenge for free radicals. They are active against a wide variety of oxidants and free radicals. Different bioflavonoids should be used for specific conditions. Bioflavonoids are found in the soft white portion between the outer rind and pulp of citrus fruits. Some are also present in grains like buckwheat and in most fruits and vegetables. Onions and garlic also contain bioflavonoids.

Milk Thistle: Milk thistle has flavonoid molecules with a strong affinity for the liver. Another example, Ginkgo biloba extract, increases general health in the elderly. Many common complaints of the elderly are a result of insuffi-

What a wonderful life I've had!
I only wish I'd realized it sooner.

Colette (1873 - 1954)

cient blood and oxygen supply. Ginkgo biloba extract has demonstrated remarkable effects in improving blood and oxygen supply to tissues. The best way to ensure an adequate intake of flavonoids is to eat a varied diet rich in fruits and vegetables.

For Better Sight

Once again, it's antioxidants to the rescue. Macular degeneration is a thinning of the macula (a part of the retina) that is the most common cause of blindness in the elderly. In a study conducted at the Massachusetts Eye and Ear Infirmary, ophthalmologist Johanna Seddon discovered that patients eating antioxidant-rich fruits and vegetables reduced their risk of this disease by half. And it was spinach that appeared to provide the most effective protection.

Seddon maintains that two of the antioxidants present in leafy greens (try collards and kale as well as spinach) also appear to block out blue light which is damaging to the retina.

Counterproductive Pollution and Diet

If you live in a polluted area and eat fatty foods, your body will generate a higher ratio of free radicals than is considered healthy. Today, with pollution at serious levels at many locations around the world, it has become more difficult to preserve a lifestyle free of the damaging effects of pollution. It is wise to consume a sufficient level of antioxidants to combat these circumstances. Some will require more than others depending on their environmental and lifestyle concerns.

Supplements, Pro and Con

Linus Pauling, a scientist and Nobel Prize winner, has written: "My estimate, made on the basis of the results of epidemiological studies, is that through the optimum use of vitamin supplements and other health measures, the length of life and well-being could be increased by 25 to 35 years."

I know many older people and several younger ones who swear by their programs of vitamin and mineral supplementation. Numerous people have told me that after many years of taking vitamin supplements, they stopped due to concerns voiced in the media, but went back to their supplements

It is a very wonderful thing about life:
if you refuse to accept anything but the best
you very often get it.

W. Somerset Maugham (1874 - 1965)

because they simply did not feel well without them. They were convinced that vitamin and mineral supplements were keeping them healthy and active.

When I was pregnant, I had the same reaction when I stopped taking my vitamins and minerals. I ran out of my supply while I was traveling and didn't bother to refill them until nearly a month had passed. I remember I had less energy and one of my teeth started to loosen. After a few days of taking supplements again, the tooth felt firm in its socket and I had my usual energy back.

I believe supplements are most important when, as a result of inferior diet, your body is not receiving the nutrients it needs. Also, when you are under a great deal of stress, in poor health or pregnant, your body seems to need more vitamins and minerals. I buy mine in a natural food store so I can be sure they come from natural food sources. I do not want to consume synthetic vitamins or artificial ingredients like fillers and binders. **It is advised that anyone who desires to begin a specific vitamin or mineral therapy should consult with a health professional first.**

Cut Calories, Add Years

There are studies that suggest cutting your caloric intake may add years to your life. A study conducted by the National Institute of Aging put rhesus and squirrel monkeys on a diet containing two-thirds of the calories fed to a control group of monkeys. After four years of calorie cutting, the leaner monkeys were healthier and aging more slowly than the "well-fed" groups. It is not certain whether this means thinner primates age slower, but it certainly suggests this possibility.

My personal opinion on this is that there is a great deal of truth in the suggestion that those who eat and drink less age more slowly. I have on occasion dramatically decreased my food intake, and it has always made me feel much better. I have more energy and vitality during these intervals. I need less sleep, my skin looks more radiant, and my digestion works better. If I have a physical problem, like a cold sore or a pain somewhere, it seems to heal more quickly when I cut down on my calories. I also focus better, think with greater clarity and accomplish more.

My personal experience has shown me that too much food slows down my body functions. It makes me sluggish and weary and seems to rob me of energy. If you are ill, overeating may inhibit your healing. Eating a lot of food also keeps you fat and prevents you from attaining your ideal weight.

Herbs

Many of the problems associated with aging have to do with a decline in the

A good Kitchen
is a good Apothecaries shop.

William Bullein (d. 1576)

body's mechanical abilities. Joints suffer fatigue from a lifetime of wear and tear. The digestive system rebels from lack of healthy fiber. Even the mind can grow lazy from lack of adequate stimulation. Herbs provide a worthy source of natural medicines to support the body's natural functions. A decline in vital energy—a frequent complaint of many past middle age—can be mitigated through the practical use of herbs. Of course, any herbal treatment is most effective when coupled with a healthy diet and lifestyle. If you take herbs to enhance your immune system but still eat unhealthy foods or live an unhealthy lifestyle, the effectiveness of herbal supplements will be diminished.

Herbs have many benefits associated with alleviating symptoms we associate with aging. They help cleanse and purify the body. They also help regulate and tone the glands to support efficient function. Herbs are high in vitamins, minerals and other necessary nutrients. Most important, herbs stimulate the body's immune system.

Herbs are classified by the Food and Drug Administration (FDA) as foods—not drugs. However, if you are not familiar with herbs at all and have no knowledge about their effect on your health, I strongly suggest that you seek the advice of your physician or herbalist. Some herbs have toxic properties when taken in excess amounts over a prolonged period of time—so please exercise caution!

Don't Wait to Lose Weight

Waiting till your next New Year's resolution to shed those extra pounds? You might want to reconsider. A study at Johns Hopkins Medical School found that additional weight carried in early life was likely to contribute to osteoarthritis further down the road. Even ten extra pounds can damage the shock-absorbing cartilage that cushions the space between weight-bearing bones. There's no time like the present for weight loss.

Diet and Lifestyle

Let's consider the eating habits of the majority of people in this country: overeating; eating "on the run"; choosing the wrong foods; consuming a lot of refined grains; failing to eliminate salt, sugar, chemical preservatives, additives, flavors and colorings from the diet. Not a pretty picture.

Now let's look at the typical American's lifestyle: lack of exercise, stress,

An Herbal Sampler

Your local health food store is likely to stock these herbs.

Alfalfa Use leaves, petals, flowers and sprouts. Detoxifies the liver. Good for colon disorders.

Astragalus Use roots as a diuretic. Increases metabolism and promotes healing.

Bee pollen Use fresh pollen from bees to combat fatigue, depression or colon disorders.

Black cohosh Use roots to help relieve asthma and sinusitis. Reduces mucus levels and can be helpful in treating high cholesterol and high blood pressure.

Blue vervain Use roots, leaves and stems to treat cold or fever. Excellent aid in expelling phlegm from throat and chest.

Butcher's broom Use tops and seeds for leg cramps, varicose veins, and circulatory disorders.

Celery seed Use juice, roots and seeds to reduce blood pressure. Acts as a sedative.

Chamomile Use flower as sleep aid and nerve tonic. An effective digestive aid.

Dong qui Use roots to treat symptoms of PMS and menopausal problems such as hot flashes and vaginal dryness.

Echinacea Use roots and leaves to boost immune system. Has antibiotic and antiviral properties.

Flax seed Use seeds to treat colon problems. Promotes strong teeth, nails and bones.

Garlic Use bulb for its natural antibiotic properties. Helpful in the treatment of arteriosclerosis, asthma and infections.

Ginseng Use roots to promote lung function, enhance immune function and normalize blood pressure.

Horehound Use flowers and leaves to treat coughs. Decreases thickness of mucus.

Licorice root Use this root to treat hypoglycemia, colitis, colds and nausea.

Mullein Use leaves as a pain killer and sleep aid. Useful in treating warts.

Parsley Use the whole plant as a diuretic. Excellent in treatment of indigestion, fluid retention and menstrual problems.

Psyllium Use seeds as a stool softener. Prevents constipation and cleans intestines.

Red raspberry Use bark, leaves and roots for strengthening uterine walls. Decreases menstrual bleeding and aids in the healing of canker sores.

Slippery elm Use inner bark to help cure diarrhea and soothe inflamed mucous membranes of the stomach, bowels and urinary tract.

Uva ursi Use leaves to combat bladder infections and kidney stones. An excellent diuretic.

White oak bark Use bark to treat PMS, varicose veins, kidney stones, gallstones and bladder problems.

Yerbamite Use all parts to treat arthritis, fluid retention and hemorrhoids. A powerful blood cleanser.

It is important to recognize that the metabolism of elderly people is frequently slowed down. Doses for people in their seventies or eighties may be lower than what is appropriate for those in their forties.

worry, lack of sleep or inability to sleep soundly, overwork, emotional mood swing, and living in a polluted area. How dreadful to realize that the richest nation in the world is failing to endorse a healthier life for its citizens. Careless eating and an unhealthful lifestyle weaken your immune system by putting stress on your body and lowering its resistance, thereby effectively shortening your life span.

While I have written in detail about the importance of colon cleansing, I want to stress once more the value of home enemas, colon hydrotherapy and diet in slowing down the aging process, particularly for women who are middle aged and older. Keep in mind that cultured and fermented dairy products are easier to digest than regular milk and cheese. They also contain lactobacteria, which are beneficial to the intestinal tract. Cultured dairy foods include yogurt, buttermilk and cottage cheese. Remember to eat lots of fruits and vegetables, sprouted whole grains, beans and dried peas, raw nuts and seeds. These foods contain a balance of vitamins, minerals, natural oils, carbohydrates and proteins. They are also high in dietary fiber.

Dietary Fiber

Dietary fiber is material from plant cells that humans cannot digest or can only partially digest. A diet high in fiber moves food through the system quickly and reduces the contact time between harmful carcinogens and intestinal tissue. It is recommended that you take in up to thirty-five grams of fiber each day. Unfortunately, most people consume only about eleven grams of fiber daily. Modern environmental pollutants expose us to a great many carcinogens. The longer waste materials remain in the body, the greater the risk that cells will absorb the poisons and become cancerous. "You are what you absorb from what you eat" might be a good way of describing it.

When you prepare your food, it is a good idea to provide yourself with fruits, vegetables, beans, peas and grains in large quantities so you will have plenty of leftovers. When high-fiber foods are readily available, they are more likely to be included in meals. That way, you will not be tempted to cook other foods which are lower in fiber.

There are two kinds of fiber—insoluble and soluble. Insoluble fiber is found in fruits, vegetables, wheat and rice bran. It scrubs the intestinal tract lining and can prevent constipation and other digestive problems, including colon cancer. Soluble fiber is found in fruits, oats and oat bran, rice bran, dried peas and beans. It swells in the presence of liquids and is thought to lower blood cholesterol and the low-density lipoproteins that carry cholesterol through the blood.

Physical activity deters disease,
while the absence of exercise encourages it.

In America, the demand for laxatives has generated business to the tune of $750 million each year. What does it say about our dietary habits when the production and sale of laxatives is a multi-million dollar-business? Clearly, it is time to move away from a diet of processed starchy, fatty and sugary foods to one high in dietary fiber. Ample fiber in our diets may prove disastrous to the laxative industry, but it will help us to vanquish digestive tract disorders such as appendicitis, colitis, hemorrhoids and, of course, constipation. We should also increase our liquid intake and get out there and exercise! Without a healthier lifestyle, chances for a long, happy life are reduced. Why stack the deck against your own success? Change your life for the better! Get started on a healthy regime today.

Exercise and Aging

Exercise is of great importance when it comes to keeping your colon healthy and clean. If you are seated most of the day and do not move around very much, your system probably will not eliminate its waste as efficiently as it should. Get up on your feet and move around. Walking, biking, dancing and swimming are great exercises for women of all ages. If you watch television or ride in a car for over an hour, make sure you walk around for five to ten minutes afterward to stimulate circulation.

If you park your car one mile from your office, you give yourself the opportunity to walk two miles each day. If that is too much, start block by block. Physical activity deters disease, while the absence of exercise encourages it. It is never too late to start exercising! Research shows that even people in their nineties can triple their strength and increase muscle size as much as 10% after just eight weeks of strength training. If you start an exercise program in mid-life, make sure you start slowly and increase the length and intensity of your workouts gradually. Such activity may also prove to have a relaxing effect, and it certainly will increase muscle endurance over time.

Walking is probably the easiest way to exercise. It is the ideal way for people over fifty to stay fit, and is one of the fastest growing "sports" in the country.

Managing Menopause Successfully

Fifty percent of women experience the onset of menopause between their mid-forties and age fifty. Approximately 25% go through it in their thirties, and the remaining 25% begin "the change" after they enter their fifties. Today, there are 40 million women in America in or past menopause.

Menopause marks the beginning of the end of menstruation and a woman's reproductive years. Just as the onset of menopause is subtle, its

*While our mass media continue to lavish
attention upon youth culture,
there are voices out there calling for women
to embrace their age and walk with conviction
into their futures.*

emotional symptoms can be more insinuated than precise. Anxiety about change in one's physical appearance can come and go. Irritability is frequently an understandable reaction to life's injustices. But combine these with sadness and insomnia and mood swings and you have the range of difficult emotions associated with menopause.

Many of the physical complaints are more precise. Headaches, muscle pain, hot flashes, vaginal dryness and night sweats are all very clear indicators that a woman is entering menopause. Fortunately, women are growing increasingly educated about their bodies and refusing to slip into obscurity as they enter this new chapter of their lives. We have more and more role models, from actresses to activists to politicians, who spend their postmenopausal years as vibrant, sexy, active women: committed advocates for their own fine quality of life. While our mass media continue to lavish attention upon youth culture, there are voices out there calling for women to embrace their age and walk with conviction into their futures.

What are some of the things we can do to ease the transition into menopause? Most obvious is a woman's determination to value herself as a mentor and inspiration to others in her life. Though childbearing ends, the need for wise and nurturing women is constant. Think of yourself as someone with something to offer your family and your community. Seek out literature or even support groups that can help you to understand this complex and inevitable process.

As to the physical symptoms, although it is controversial, an increasing number of gynecologists are recommending hormone replacement therapy to their menopausal patients. A recent study of 875 women at seven medical centers offers encouraging news about progesterone-estrogen hormone replacement. While estrogen therapy has shown undeniable success in combating heart disease in menopausal women, it appears to increase the risk of uterine cancer. The addition of progesterone diminished the risk of uterine cancer but was thought to cancel out the heart-protecting benefits of estrogen. This study revealed that the women taking the progesterone-estrogen combination derived the same heart disease protection as their estrogen taking counterparts. Interestingly, natural progesterone from soybeans provided the most effective benefit.

A very significant study was published in the *New England Journal of Medicine* entitled "The Use of Estrogens and Progestins and the Risk of Breast Cancer in Postmenopausal Women" (Vol. 332, p. 1559, June 15, 1995). The study followed 121,700 nurses for over twenty years and determined that hormone replacement therapy, whether estrogen alone or cou-

The key is to remain open to possibility.

pled with progesterone, did increase the incidence of breast cancer among postmenopausal women. Women taking the hormones for more than five years were found to have a 46% greater risk of developing breast cancer than women who never received the therapy. The study goes on to say that the benefits of hormone replacement therapy may outweigh the hazards for women at high risk of heart disease and osteoporosis. But for women at low risk of developing these conditions, the heightened peril of breast cancer may make hormone supplements a significant gamble. Dr. Graham A. Colditz, principal author of the study, concludes, "It clearly raises the need to reconsider risk and benefits if a woman is going to use the hormones for more than five years."

The decision to use hormone replacement therapy is one that must be made by a woman in consultation with a trusted physician. Just as we all comparison shop when making a significant purchase, we must all become informed consumers when something so precious as our health is concerned. With all of the serious implications surrounding synthetic hormone replacement, I believe we are well advised to at least consider an herbal estrogen replacement program. An increasing number of M.D.s, herbalists and homeopathic physicians are eager to work with women who wish to maximize their own body's potential to stimulate the natural production of estrogen. While it is imperative that every woman consult her health care practitioner, I can heartily recommend several fundamental steps to managing menopause successfully:

•Coffee and cigarettes deplete the body of naturally occurring estrogen—Give them up!

•Regular exercise is a postmenopausal woman's best friend. A moderate workout in the fresh air is best. Walking, jogging, tennis, swimming, cycling, golf or weightlifting will enhance your positive outlook and keep you fit.

•Cut down on fat to minimize your risk of heart disease. Make sure your are eating foods rich in vitamin E and calcium.

•Following is a list of herbs used in the management of menopause: Mexican wild yam, unicorn root, false unicorn root, elder, sarsaparilla, holy thistle, passion flower, raspberry, sage, ladyslipper.

Before starting an herbal program, be sure to consult a licensed herbalist and invest in one or two of the excellent books available on medicinal herbs.

Osteoporosis
Small-boned women of Northern European extraction, smokers and women

There are always many blessings
if you choose to look for them.

who enter menopause early are considered candidates for osteoporosis. A lifelong commitment to exercise is the best defense against this bone-weakening disease. A diet high in calcium is also imperative. To enhance your ability to absorb calcium, eat foods high in vitamin D and be sure to get plenty of sunshine. Cut back on alcohol, salt, sugar and animal protein, all of which rob you of the calcium you have worked so hard to preserve.

Attitude and Aging

Please remind yourself frequently to keep a positive, constructive, joyous outlook on life. View life as a cup half full, not half empty. Every day, thank God for everything you have to be grateful for in your life. There are always many blessings if you choose to look for them. Focus on what you have and what you can do rather than emphasizing what you lack and cannot accomplish right away. Stay loving, and forgive shortcomings in the people you meet.

It is so important to stay physically and mentally active all of your life. Get involved in outside activities and meet new people. Remember, there is only one "you" in this world. You are totally special and different from everyone else. Value yourself and everyone you meet. There is no way of predicting when you're going to meet someone who will greatly enrich your life. The key is to remain open to possibility. Look for the good and emphasize it. You have unique contributions to make to the world. No one else can do exactly what you do. Identify and develop your own special talents. Work to grow spiritually and give all you can. The more you give, the more will come back to you. Never let your chronological age stop you from doing what you want to do or changing old habits. Just as you are what you eat, so you also are as young (or as old) as you feel. Remember, it's never too late to live your life fully!

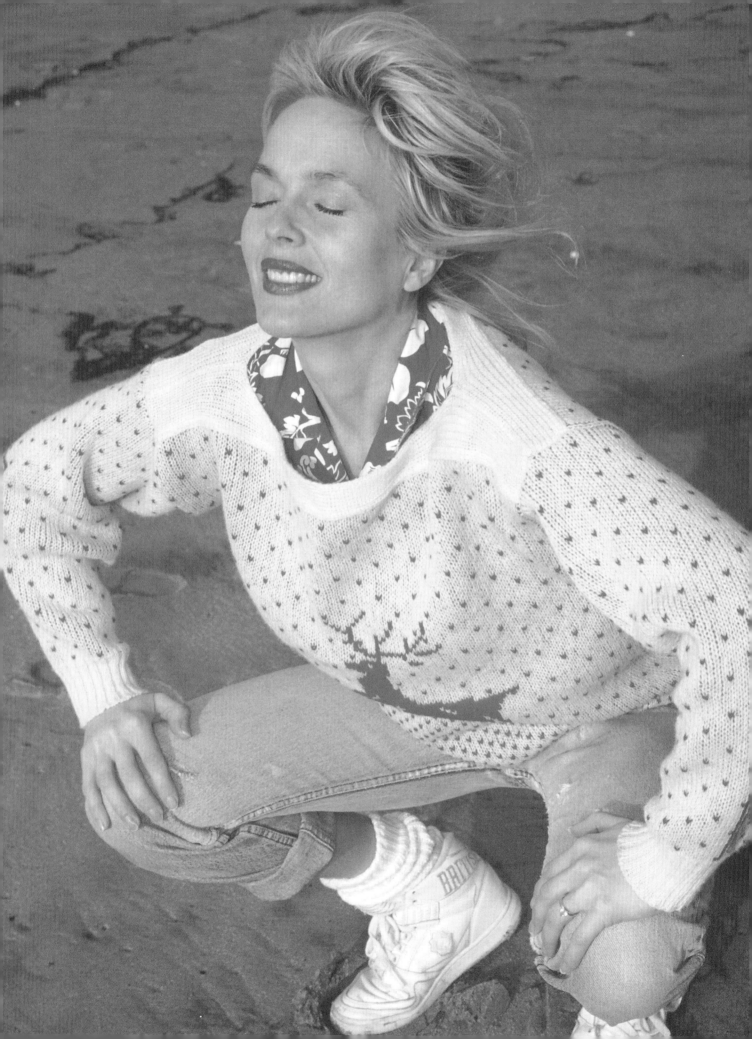

CHAPTER TEN

Thinking, Spirituality and Attitude

It is very important to recognize that mind and body work together. You must do your best to keep your thoughts high and pure at the same time that you discipline your body to function at peak efficiency. Your state of mind is very important if you want to look and feel your best. Good food choices make you feel so great that your attitude cannot help but improve. With a joyous, positive mental attitude and a clean, strong body, you become the best you can be. With commitment, you can develop your talents to their fullest potential. The road is open for each of us to achieve our highest goals and our most challenging dreams.

The mind exerts its powerful influence over the body, just as the state of the body influences the mind. Therefore, a clean, pure bloodstream is essential to clean, pure thoughts. Anxiety and depression affect the body by releasing

You will always be truly beautiful
in mind and body if you invest all your time
being the best you can be to yourself
and your fellow human beings.

digestive juices and secretions which can cause ulcers and literally eat out your insides. When you are happy and excited, your body releases endorphins which make you feel good. Endorphins replicate energy that is not unlike the rush of adrenaline experienced in times of stress. It is also easier to exercise and reject the temptation to eat "junk foods" when you are in a positive frame of mind.

I believe in being the best you can be in all areas of your life. Set goals and work to achieve them. That is the only way you will realize true happiness. When you are aware of your power and express it productively, you cannot help but radiate true beauty. Everyone will be drawn to you, and you will be a winner in the true sense of the word.

When I look back on my life, I review all the positive changes I have made. I consider myself lucky to have been born with the potential for physical good looks. Until several years ago, however, I had not developed my potential for higher spiritual living and a pure and healthy body. I was in my twenties when I first became curious about those aspects of life.

Now I look at my photographs from that time period and see that I have gained a more pure and refined beauty since educating myself about spiritual matters. Today there is much more joy and love and even fun in my eyes. Instead of becoming less beautiful as I have grown older, I feel I have grown more youthful.

People who have not seen me for many years often comment on this, and no stranger ever succeeds in guessing my chronological age. Most people guess I am at least ten years younger than I am. I believe that this is my reward for learning lessons in self-care and positive thinking. I intend to go on developing and educating myself in mind and body so that I can become the best person I can be. I want my life to be an example to others and I want to share my wisdom with them.

Education and Discipline

As we age, there is an unnatural tendency to grow unhealthier in mind and body. It is up to each one of us to discipline ourselves toward superior health and happiness by living and thinking correctly. You are as old as you feel, and if you are living right, you will not "grow old" as the years pass by. Years have nothing to do with aging. They are simply road signs for the passing of time. One can be "old" at age 25 or "young" at 75.

The condition of your body is a direct result of the mental and physical care it has received over time. Mental care is of prime importance. Many people seem to forget to take care of their mental state. Some become pre-

For beauty being the best of all we know

sums up the unsearchable

and secret aims of nature.

Robert Bridges (1844 - 1930) British poet

occupied with athletic workouts and change themselves with plastic surgery. No matter how physically perfect they look on the outside, it is a mistake for anyone to neglect the importance of his or her state of mind. In the long run, the way you think will make or break you. That's why first and foremost, you must give special time and attention to taking control of your thoughts. If you constantly worry about potential ailments and sickness, you will never be healthy. You cannot be happy if you continuously think negative, depressing and destructive thoughts. If you want to feel great and be beautiful, you must not wrap yourself in the cloak of fear of old age.

Positive Thinking

To remain young and truly beautiful in spirit, put all your efforts into gaining the enduring attributes of youth and beauty: energy, vitality, good health and joy. This means being loving, giving, compassionate, genial, cordial, polite and understanding to everyone you encounter in your life.

You must also remain productive and creative and spend your time wisely. There should never be a time when you cannot figure out what to do with yourself. Expand and use your imagination. There is so much you can do. You possess enough power and talent to tackle any project you wish. The only one who can stop you from succeeding in your life is you.

You are your own enemy if you allow negative and fearful thoughts to rule your actions. Think about it every day and choose to replace every negative thought that crosses your mind with a more powerful positive one. Concentrate on being constructive. Encourage, inspire and give to others as well as yourself each day and count that day a success. Never be afraid of giving. The more you give, the more you will have.

You will always be truly beautiful in mind and body if you invest all your time being the best you can be to yourself and your fellow human beings. It takes a huge amount of determination and commitment to spend your life in this positive manner, but what other alternative do we have? If you fail to take charge and follow this path, you will probably become weaker mentally, deteriorate physically, lose your beauty, and get old before your time. Is that where you want life to lead you?

If you develop yourself into the best that you can be, you will get so much more out of life. There are no limitations on how far you can go and how much you can achieve. Nothing can stop you once you decide to achieve a well-thought-out goal.

The body must be repaired and supported,
if we would preserve
the mind in all its vigour.

Pliny the Younger (62 AD - 113 AD) Roman Politician

Productive Lifetime

When you are 80 years of age, wouldn't it be wonderful to be in superior health and as productive and youthful—even as beautiful—as ever before in your life? I certainly think so. I do not intend to become old and sick and watch myself fade away. I would rather do the work it takes to continue being the best I can be for as long as I live. Think of how much more you can contribute to the world that way. Adopt your very own mission in life and give something back. Think of how much God gave you. It is a debt of tremendous proportion and requires that you give back all you can. It is actually easier to contribute to society at large after you have educated and developed your own mind and body to their highest potential.

First of all, from the minute I wake up, I take hold of my thinking to keep it positive and constructive. Fear is a tricky adversary and sometimes it takes great discipline to banish it from your heart. I believe in God, and ask each day for strength and guidance and protection against all evil. In the past, I spent many days being depressed, destructive and filled with fear. Sometimes those same negative influences still creep up on me and almost take over. Now I can consciously grab hold of myself and rid my mind of such thoughts. This is a battle which I face nearly every day, but I remain peaceful, productive and constructive most of the time because I have learned to control my thinking.

Always See Beauty

The person who continues to see beauty in everything will always be young. It is important to perceive beauty in your world throughout life. That is one of the most valuable tools in remaining vital and young at heart. Age does not make you ugly. When you can look in the mirror and value the image looking back at you, then you are seeing beyond superficial beauty to true beauty. Inner beauty is timeless beauty. Its building blocks are positive thoughts, joy, industry, optimism and courage. This beauty that shines from the eyes of loving people is strong and compelling and will never fade.

Don't fight with yourself about aging. Don't hate yourself a little more every time you detect a little sag or wrinkle or an ache or pain that was absent before. Don't regard each minute detail as a defeat in life. That kind of criticism shows the worst disrespect to the self.

I want to make aging a positive experience, not a negative one. You can too. Let's do all the things we can do to stay healthy, youthful, beautiful and productive for as long as we live. When we make our best effort in life, we feel the most fulfilled for having done so.

Suggested Readings

Back to Eden: The Classic Guide to Herbal Medicine, Natural Foods and Home Remedies, Kloss, Woodridge Press Publishing Comp., 1972

Mucusless-Diet Healing System, Arnold Ehret, Lust, 1976

Thus Speaketh the Stomach (Also The Tragedy of Nutrition), Arnold Ehret, Ehret Literature, 1977

The Definite Cure of Constant Constipation, Arnold Ehret, Lust, 1983

Be Your Own Doctor: A Positive Guide to Natural Healing, Ann Wigmore, Avery Publ., 1982

The Hippocrates Diet and Health Program, Ann Wigmore, Avery Publ., 1984

Why Suffer?, Ann Wigmore, Avery Publ., 1985

Recipes for Longer Life, Ann Wigmore, Avery Publ., 1978

The Healing Power Within: Tapping the Infinite Potential from Within Yourself, Ann Wigmore, Avery Publ., 1983

The Grapevine, Johanna Brandt, Lust, 1971

Diet for a New America: How Your Food Choices Effect Your Health, Happiness and the Future of Life on Earth, John Robbins, Still Point Publ., 1992

Diet for a New World: May All be Fed, John Robbins, Morrow, 1992

Become Younger, N.W. Walker, O'Sullivan Woodside Co., 1975

Fresh Vegetable and Fruit Juices: What's Missing in Your Body, N.W. Walker, Norwalk Press, 1970

Diet & Salad: The Vegetarian Guide To, N.W. Walker, Norwalk Press, 1971

Vegetarian Baby: A Complete and Valuable Sourcebook for Vegetarian Parents, Sharon Yutema, MC Books Press, 1984

Vibrant Health: The Natural Way To, N.W. Walker, Norwalk Press, 1977

Colon Health: Key to a Vibrant Life, N.W. Walker, Norwalk Press, 1979

How to Get Well: Dr. Ariola's Handbook of Natural Healing, Paavo Ariola, Health Plus Publ., 1974

How to Keep Slim, Healthy, and Young with Juice Fasting, Paavo Ariola, Health Plus Publ., 1971

Fasting Can Save Your Life, Herbert Shelton, Natural Hygiene, 1981

Science and Fine Art of Food and Nutrition, Herbert Shelton, Natural Hygiene, 1984

Food Combining Made Easy, Herbert Shelton, Natural Hygiene, 1982

Food and Healing, Anne Marie Colbin, Ballantine Books, 1986

The Book of Whole Meals: A Seasonal Guide to Assembling Balanced Vegetarian Breakfasts, Lunches and Dinners, Anne Marie Colbin, Ballantine Books, 1985

Transition for Vegetarianism: An Evolutionary Step, Rudolf Ballantine, Himalayan Publ., 1987

Diet for a Small Planet, France Moore Lappe, Ballantine Books, 1991

The Colon Health Handbook, Robert Gray, Emerald Publ., 1980

You Can Waste Disease: What You Need to Know, Prevention of Disease Our Goal, Bernard Feasen, Bernard Feasen Publ. Div., 1984

Tissue Cleansing Through Bowel Management: With the Ultimate Tissue Cleansing System, Bernard Feasen & Sylvia Bell, Bernard Feasen Enterprises, 1981

Index

Acid-alkaline connection, 85-87

Aging
education and discipline, 227-229
and a productive lifetime, 231
seeing beauty in everything, 231

Aging reversal, 201-223
antioxidant compounds, 205-209
antioxidants and free radicals, 203-205
attitude and aging, 223
counterproductive pollution and diet, 209
cutting calories and adding years, 211
diet and lifestyle, 213-215
dietary fiber, 215-217
estrogen usage, 219-221
exercise and aging, 217
herbs, 211-213
hormone replacement therapy, 219-221
list of herbs, 214
losing weight, 213
macular degeneration, 209
menopause management, 217-221
osteoporosis, 221-223
phytochemicals, 205
research on aging, 203
supplements, 209-211
Alliance of Family Farmers, 57
Aloe vera, 175, 191
Americans, fat sources consumed by, 91
Amiel, Henri, 138
Antioxidants
compounds, 205-209
and free radicals, 203-205
Aspertame debate, 49

Baking vegetables, 71
Baths, seaweed, 185-187
Beauty
inner, 231
seeing, 231
Beauty tips, timeless, 171-199
basic reminders, 195-197
deep breathing exercise, 173-175
dental hygiene, 183
guided imagery, 173
hair care, 187-189
lemon wedges, 191
magical mystery paste, 183
make-up, 183-185
masks, 185
meditation, 171-173
minimizing jet lag, 195
protection from the sun, 189-191
relaxation, 197-199
relief for aching muscles, 187
sea kelp, 193
sea salt, 193
seaweed, 191
seaweed baths, 185-187
skin care, 175-177
aloe vera, 175
calendula cream, 175
dry brushing, 177-179
wet cleansing, 179-181
slant board, 181
sunscreens, 191
sunshine, 177
tea tree oil (*melaleuca alternifolia*), 193
travel tips, 193-195

Biggs, Hermann M., 15
Blake, William, 198
Breads, whole grain, 41-43
Breakfasts, 151
Breathing exercises, deep, 173-175
Bridges, Robert, 228
Brillat-Savarin, Anthelme, 34
Bug repellant, homemade, 57
Bullein, William, 212
Bulletin of the New York Academy of Medicine, 28
C. Everett Koop Foundation, 67
Calendula cream, 175
Calories, cutting, 211
Carbohydrates
    recommended, 71
    and sugars, 67
Charts
    exercise - workout - benefits, 169
    food combining, 75
    healthy eating, 35
    suggested foods, 44-45

Chinese cooking, 43
Cholesterol
    and fat, 89-91
      high density lipoproteins (HDLs), 89
      low density lipoproteins (LDLs), 89

Cicero, Marcus Tullius, 48, 144
Cleobulus, 22, 64
Colditz, Graham A., 221
Colette, 208
Comfort foods, 27
Constipation relief, 159
Cooking
Chinese, 43
    tips, 81
Cravings, food, 31

Delicious Magazine, 189
Dental hygiene, 183
Descartes, René, 143
Diarrhea relief, 159
Dietary fibers, 215-217
Diets
    directions, 31-37
    and health, 83-103
    and lifestyle, 213-215
    mono, 153
    mucus free, 99-103
    raw vegetarian, 23
    vegetarian, 87
Digestion, salads aid, 65
Dr. Jensen's Dry Vegetable Seasoning, 25

Eating meat, 47
Eggless Egg Salad, 87
Emerson, Ralph Waldo, 172
Endorphins defined, 143
Energy and holistic health, 143
Energy soup, 113
Environmental Protection Agency (EPA), 55
Estrogen usage, 219-221
Exercise
    and aging, 217
    auxiliary benefits, 167-169
    benefits circulation, 167
    a daily routine, 163
    deep breathing, 173-175
    and fitness, 161-169
    revitalization of the body, 161-163
    routine, 165-167
    workout - benefits chart, 169
    workout at home, 165
    workout in the gym, 165

Fasting
    alternatives, 151-153

effects, 145

eliminating toxins, 147-149

extended juice fast, 149-151

heightened healing, 147

help with medical problems, 145-147

and holistic health, 143-153

no breakfast, no junk foods, 151

sense of taste, 147

Fatigue and excess weight, 67-69

Fats

and cholesterol, 89-91

recommended, 73

sources consumed by Americans, 91

Fiber, dietary, 215-217

Fitness and exercise, 161-169

Food choices

alternatives, 27

author's personal program, 25-29

author's philosophy, 21-25

cravings, 31

diet directions, 31-37

eating different foods, 29-31

eating meat, 47

exotic grains, 41-43

fresh fruits/vegetables, 47-49

health and happiness, 29

healthy, 19-57

healthy eating chart, 35

healthy snacking, 37

observations, 29-31

protein rich foods, 43, 47

protein rich foods and water, 47

snack alternatives, 33

sodas, 39

successful snacking, 37

suggested foods chart, 44-45

sweet alternatives, 37-40

vegetarianism, 53-55

whole grain breads and pastas, 41-43

Food and Drug Administration (FDA), 51, 213

Foods

chart, 44-45

comfort, 27

junk, 37, 151, 227

menus, 76-79

organically grown, 55-57

and pesticides, 55-57

protein-rich, 43

suggested, 44-45

to avoid, 49-53

Foods, combining, 59-81

basic food types, 61-63

carbohydrates and sugars, 67

chart, 75

cooking tips, 81

examples, 69-71

excess weight and fatigue, 67-69

a new system, 63

recommended carbohydrates, 71

recommended fats, 73

recommended proteins, 73

recommended salad ingredients, 71

recommended vegetables for steaming

and baking, 71

rules, 65

salads aid digestion, 65

words of encouragement, 73-81

Free radicals, 203-205

Fruits

fresh vegetables and, 47-49

recipes, 117

sorbets (home preparation), 111-113

Grains

exotic, 41-43

and health, 87

Guided imagery, 173

Hair care, 187-189
Healing and fasting, 147
Health
      holistic, 137-159
      neglecting one's, 15
      perspectives, 14
Health and diet, 83-103
      acid-alkaline connection, 85-87
      cholesterol and fat, 89-91
      cow's milk and milk products, 91-93
      Eggless Egg Salad, 87
      and grains, 87
      meat and other proteins, 83-85
      and mucus, 99-101
      mucus free diet, 99-103
      refined sugar, 97-99
      salt, 93-97
      salt and herbs, 95
      sugarless and sugar-free products, 97-99
      vegetarian diet benefits, 87
Healthy eating chart, 35
Herbs, 211-213
      list of, 214
      and salt, 95
Hippocrates, 140
Holistic health, 137-159
      analyzing iris of the eye, 153
      awakenings, 139-141
      constipation relief, 159
      diarrhea relief, 159
      and energy, 143
      and fasting, 143-153
      fasting alternatives, 151-153
      effects, 145
      eliminating toxins, 147-149
      extended juice fast, 149-151
      heightened healing, 147
      help with medical problems, 145-147
      no breakfast, no junk foods, 151

      sense of taste, 147
      foods which support life, 141-143
      internal cleansing, 153-155
      colon controversies, 155
      home enema program, 157-159
      iridology, 153
      learning to eat right, 137-139
      natural health practices, 155-157
      water - first step to a healthy lifestyle, 141
Hormone replacement therapy, 219-221
Hygiene, dental, 183

Illnesses, prevention of, 63
Imagery, guided, 173
Iridology defined, 153
Iris (of the eye), 153

Jet lag, minimizing, 195
John Hopkins Medial School, 213
Juices
      extended fasts, 149-151
      smoothies, shakes & sorbets, 105-111
Junk foods, 37, 151, 227

Kelp, sea, 193

Labels, "certified organic", 55
Lifetime, productive, 231

Macular degeneration, 209
Make-up, 183-185
Masks, 185
Maugham, W. Somerset, 210
Meat, eating, 47
Meat and other proteins, 83-85
Meditation, 171-173
Menopause management, 217-221
Menus, 76-79
Milk and milk products, 91-93

Mono diet, 153
Movie stars, American, 13
Mucus
    free diet, 99-103
    and fruits and vegetables, 99
    and health, 99-101
Munro, Hector Hugh, 176
Murray, Michael, 203
Muscles, relief for aching, 187

National Institute of Aging, 211
National Organic Directory, 57
National Pesticide Telecommunications Network, 57
Natural Health Clinic of Los Angeles, 157
"Natural" products and the FDA, 51
New England Journal of Medicine, 219
New York Obesity Research Center, 67
Nietzsche, Friedrich, 186
Nutrition components, 16
    effects of mucus-producing foods, 16
    importance of food combinations, 16
    type of food/fuel consumed, 16

Oil, tea tree, 193
Organic vegetables, 57
Osler, William, 162
Osteoporosis, 221-223
Ozone, 167

Pastas, 41-43
Pauling, Linus, 209
Pesticides
    and food, 55-57
        National Pesticide Telecommunications
Network, 57
Phytochemicals, 205
Picasso, Pablo, 204
Pizzorno, Joseph, 203

Playboy magazine, 14
Pliny the Younger, 230
Pregnancy, 119-135
    daily hygiene, 123
    diet, 123-125
    cravings, 127-129
    eating observations, 129-131
    food favorites, 127
    increased need from protein, 125-127
    problems, 125
    resuming a normal diet after binging,
131-133
    tips, 133-135
    vitamin/mineral supplements, 129
    exercising body and mind, 121-123
    general impressions, 133
Progesterone, 219
Progestins, 219
Protein rich foods, 43, 47
Proteins
    and meat, 83-85
    recommended, 73

Raw vegetarian diets, 23
Recipes, 105-117
    fruit sorbets (home preparation), 111-113
    fruits, 117
    juices, smoothies, shakes & sorbets,
105-111
    veggies, soups, sandwiches, stews, 113-115
Relaxation, 197-199
Rubinstein, Helena, 194

Saki (Hector Hugh Munro), 176
Salads
    aid digestion, 65
    eggless egg, 87
    recommended ingredients, 71
Salt, 93-97

replacements, 95
sea, 193
Sandwiches, 23, 113-115
Sea kelp, 193
Sea salt, 193
Seasoning, Dr. Jensen's Dry Vegetable, 25
Seaweed, 191
Seaweed baths, 185-187
Shakes, 105-111
Shenstone, William, 178
Singer, Isaac Bashevis, 32
Skin care, 175-177
    aloe vera, 175
    calendula cream, 175
    dry brushing, 177-179
    wet cleansing, 179-181
Slant board, 181
Smith, Sydney, 60
Smog, 167
Smoothies, 105-111
Snacks
    alternatives, 33
    healthy, 37
    successful, 37
Sodas, 39
Sorbets, 105-113
Soups, 113-115
Stanley, Edward, 164
Steaming vegetables, 71
Stews, 113-115
Sugarless and sugar-free products, 97-99
Sugars
    and carbohydrates, 67
    refined, 97-99
Sullivan, Terrence, 155-157
Sun, protection from, 188
Sunscreens, 191
Sunshine, 177
Sweets, alternatives, 37-40

Tea tree oil (*melaleuca alternifolia*), 193
Theroux, Paul, 192
Thinking
    positive, 229
    spirituality and attitude, 225-231
Toxic wastes, 23
Toxins, eliminating, 147-149
Travel tips, 193-195
Tucker, Sophie, 202
Turkey, noble, 47

Vegetables
    fresh fruits and, 47-49
    organic, 57
    for steaming and baking, 71
Vegetarian diets
    benefits, 87
    raw, 23
Vegetarian sandwich, 23
Vegetarianism, 53-55
Veggies, soups, sandwiches, stews, 113-115

Wastes, toxic, 23
Water
    first step to a healthy lifestyle, 141
    and protein rich foods, 47
    recommended eight glasses per day, 141
Weight, losing, 213
Welch, Raquel, 13
Weng, Chu Hui, 28
Wheeler, Hugh, 182
Whole grain breads, 41-43
Wilde, Oscar, 126

Yutang, Lin, 40